TAI CHI SECRETS OF THE YANG STYLE

出精於勤自奮進
功夫無息法自修

楊俊敏 先生惠存

辛巳春于中國黃山原如 楊振鐸

Refined work is accomplished through self-disciplinary diligence,
ceaseless gongfu is done through constant self-cultivation.

Tai Chi Secrets of the Yang Style

Chinese Classics • Translations • Commentary

by Dr. Yang, Jwing-Ming

YMAA Publication Center
Wolfeboro, NH USA

YMAA Publication Center, Inc.
PO Box 480
Wolfeboro, NH 03894
800-669-8892 • www.ymaa.com • info@ymaa.com

ISBN 9781886969094 (print)
ISBN 9781594395000 (ebook)
ISBN 9781594394188 (hardcover)

Cover design by Katya Popova
Photos provided by the authors unless otherwise indicated.
Edited by James O'Leary

20240126

Publisher's Cataloging in Publication

(Prepared by Quality Books Inc.)

Yang, Jwing-Ming, 1946-
     Tai chi secrets of the Yang Style : Chinese classics,
translation, commentary / Yang, Jwing-Ming. -- 1st ed.
     p. cm.
     Includes bibliographical references and index.
     ISBN: 9781886969094 (print), ISBN: 9781594395000 (ebook),
     ISBN: 9781594394188 (hardcover)

     1. Tai chi. I. Title.
GV504.Y36 2001   613.7'148
                          QBI01-201112

The author and publisher of the material are NOT RESPONSIBLE in any manner whatsoever for any injury which may occur through reading or following the instructions in this manual.
The activities physical or otherwise, described in this manual may be too strenuous or dangerous for some people, and the reader(s) should consult a physician before engaging in them.
Nothing in this document constitutes a legal opinion nor should any of its contents be treated as such. While the authors believe that everything herein is accurate, any questions regarding specific self-defense situations, legal liability, and/or interpretation of federal, state, or local laws should always be addressed by an attorney at law.
When it comes to martial arts, self-defense, and related topics, no text, no matter how well written, can substitute for professional, hands-on instruction. **These materials should be used for academic study only.**

Printed in USA.

Contents

前言

任何一種體育項目，普遍來說都是在一定文化環境下產生的，都有一定的文化特徵。中國的武術亦是如此，它是以中國的傳統文化為理論基礎，受中國傳統文化環境性的影響，中國的武術家就是用中國文化去規範拳技，闡明拳理，形成文、武交融一體。尋求武術的理論，是用以指導武術的技法原理。武術的教學原則、武術的訓練原則、以及具體的拳械技法和教學訓練法等等，都體現中國傳統文化與武術運動規律的融合。比如，在武術理論中，武術技法原理強調“內外合一”；武術教學原則強調“內外兼修”；武術訓練原則強調“內外互導”。在具體的拳械動作標準中，講究“三尖相照”、“內外六合”、“五合三催”等，使動作體現出外形和諧、內意充實、形神兼備的形態。這無疑是中國傳統文化強調“天人合一”的宇宙觀，並以此來處理內與外的關係的實際例子。毫無疑問，太極拳也不例外。

正如每個人都清楚，太極拳是中國傳統武術的主要拳種之一，如上所說，太極拳就是依中國的“太極圖說”以為立論。我在楊俊敏博士的另一本譯著新書《太極拳武、李氏先哲秘要》所寫的序中曾經提過，太極拳始見自清初傳於中國河南省溫縣陳家溝，而就在這一族一地的小範圍能傳向全國，傳向世界，由陳氏太極拳一個流派發展為與其特點有異的楊氏、孫氏、吳氏、傳（振嵩）氏等等多種太極拳流派，並成為學練者最為普及的拳種，這就是太極拳不斷前進和創新的見證，而楊氏太極拳，則是從陳氏太極拳始的最早創新的鼻祖。它創自河北省永年人楊福魁（字露禪）（一七九九－一八七二年），而楊最早是師從陳家溝太極拳師陳長興為徒的。楊得傳後，於一八五零年左右返回家鄉，後被薦至北京，任京師旗營武術教師，他為了擴大傳習範圍，並適應清朝“玉體不動”的顯貴達官和體弱年邁者的體質，適應保健需要，刪改陳氏太極拳老架中的發勁、跳躍和難度較高的動作，創編成楊氏太極拳架，後又經其子楊健候（一八三九－一九一七年），其孫楊澄甫（一八三－一九三六年）等人修潤，定型為現在的楊氏太極拳套路。

楊氏太極拳動作姿勢舒展簡潔，動作鬆柔，緩慢勻速，這些亦同樣與中國古代哲學家老子的“重柔主靜”的思想相通。楊澄甫將楊氏太極拳的技法總結為十要，即：“虛靈頂勁，含胸拔背，鬆腰，分虛實，沉肩墜肘，用意不用力，上下相隨，內外相合，相連不斷，動中求靜”。而這些創新，亦均離不開以中國傳統文化的哲理去闡明。楊俊敏博士此次又收集了楊氏太極拳先哲的秘要，翻譯成書，再次以由淺入深的方法去解釋有關的哲理，其中有些是具體的楊氏太極拳各式的實用攻防技法要領；有些則是太極拳技法的哲理原由，其目的是希望中國的古老文化之一的太極拳得到發揚光大，使西方廣大愛好者能更好的理解和研習，這種奉獻的精神是難能可貴的，故再次樂而為之序。

梁強亞
二零零一年一月三十一日
於美國加州屋崙市

Foreword

Grandmaster Liang, Qiang-Ya 梁強亞

In general, any kind of physical education or training is produced from a defined culture and environment. Consequently, they all have culturally distinctive features. It is the same for Chinese Wushu (武術). The fist techniques (i.e., fighting skills) are standardized and the fist theories (i.e., fighting theories) are expounded, based on Chinese traditional culture. This results in a combined, unified body of scholarship (i.e., internal understanding) and martial arts (i.e., external manifestation). The purpose of searching for the theories of Wushu is to find instructional grounds for Wushu skills and techniques. Wushu's instructional principles and rules, Wushu's training principles and rules, and the specific fist, weapon skills and training methods, all demonstrate the blending of Chinese culture and regular Wushu athletic patterns. For example, in its theory of techniques and skills, Wushu emphasizes "the unification of internal and external" (內外合一); Wushu teaching principles stress "double cultivation of internal and external" (內外兼修); Wushu training guidelines focus on "mutual correspondence of internal and external" (內外互導). In the general standardization of the fist (i.e., barehand) and weapon's movements, it (i.e., Wushu) especially addresses "three points corresponding with each other" (三尖相照), "six harmonizations of internal and external" (內外六合), and "five unifications and three urgencies" (五合三催) etc., which therefore demonstrate its external harmonization in the movements, and enrich its internal Yi (i.e., comprehension), the state that possesses both the shape (i.e., external manifestation) and spirit (i.e., internal manifestation). This no doubt is the universal concept of "unification of the heaven and the human" (天人合一) which has been emphasized in Chinese traditional culture. Wushu is therefore a practical demonstration of the reality of this internal and external unification. There is not the slightest question that Taijiquan has these same features (i.e., traditional Chinese cultural root).

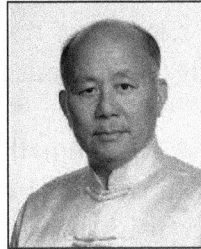

It seems clear to everyone that Taijiquan is one of the fist styles in traditional Chinese Wushu. As mentioned above, Taijiquan established its theoretical foundation on "the illustration of Taiji" (太極圖說). I have written a foreword for Dr. Yang, Jwing-Ming's other new book: *Tai Chi Secrets of Wü and Li Styles* (太極拳武、李氏先哲秘要). In this book, I mentioned that Taijiquan first spread out from Chen's village, Wen county, Henan province, China (中國・河南省・溫縣・陳家溝) at the beginning of Qing dynasty (清朝). From this small territory and clan, it spread across all of China, and now to the whole world. The styles that have developed from Chen style, and which have established their own special stylistic characteristics are: Yang (楊), Sun (孫), Wü (武), Wu (吳), and Fu (傅)(Zhen-Song)(振嵩). These well-known styles have become the most popular fist styles for many practitioners and learners. This is proof that Taijiquan has been advanced and innovated from within continuously. Yang style Taijiquan was the earliest style which was innovated from Chen Taijiquan. It was created by Yang, Fu-Kui (楊福魁)(nickname Lu-Chan)(露禪)(1799-1872) who was a disciple of Chen, Chang-Xing (陳長興) in Chen's village (陳家溝). After Yang finished his learning, he returned to his home village around 1850. Later, he was recommended to Beijing (北京) to be the Wushu teacher in the Beijing Manchurian Loyal military camp (旗營). In order to broaden the possibility of learning and also to be adopted more easily by prominent officials and eminent personages (who held the philosophy of "jade body does not move" (i.e., those who have a precious body do not work) as well as older people, for health maintenance purpose, he revised Chen Style Taijiquan Old Posture and got rid of harder actions such as Jin's emitting (Fa Jin, 發勁), jumping, and the relatively more difficult movements. Thus was created Yang Style Taijiquan. Later it was again revised and edited by his son, Yang, Jian-Hou (楊健侯)(1839-1917) and his grandson, Yang, Cheng-Fu (楊澄甫)(1883-1936), to become today's Yang Style Taijiquan routine.

The postures of Yang Style Taijiquan are comfortable, open, simple, and clear; the movements are loose, soft, slow, and uniform. These special features match the ancient Chinese philosopher Lao Zi's (老子) philosophy of "focusing the softness and maintaining the calmness" (重柔主靜). Yang, Cheng-Fu concluded that there were ten most important keys to practicing Yang Style Taijiquan skills and techniques. They are: "insubstantial energy suspends the head upward, draw in the chest and arc the back, loosen the waist, discriminate insubstantial and substantial, sink the shoulders and drop the elbows, use the Yi not the Li, top and bottom are mutually following each other, unification of internal and external, continuous without breaking, and search for calmness within movements." It cannot be denied that all of these new creations were expounded from Chinese traditional cultural philosophy.

Dr. Yang, Jwing-Ming has again collected more secrets of Yang's style and translated them into a book, and again he explains and interprets the related philosophies and theories, from the shallow to the deep. Some of them relate to the practical offensive and defensive applications of postures in Yang Style Taijiquan, and others talk about the philosophy and principles of Taijiquan skills. The purpose of all of this effort is to introduce and spread this gem of the old Chinese traditional culture, Taijiquan, to a greater number of people. Consequently, Western Taijiquan lovers will have a better opportunity to understand and study. This kind of contribution is rare and precious. Therefore, I am very happy to write this foreword for him again.

Liang, Qiang-Ya
January 31, 2001, Oakland, CA

Note: Grandmaster Liang, Qiang-Ya was born in Canton province, China in 1931. He started his Wushu training with Grandmaster Fu, Zhen-Song (1881-1953) in 1945. Grandmaster Fu, Zhen-Song was an intimate friend of Grandmasters Yang, Cheng-Fu (楊澄甫) and also Sun, Lu-Tang (孫祿堂) at the time. Consequently, the Fu Style Taijiquan (傅氏太極拳) and also Two Poles Fist (兩儀拳) created by Grandmaster Fu both blend some of the specific features of Yang and Sun Styles Taijiquan.

In addition, Grandmaster Liang, Qiang-Ya is an expert in Baguazhang and Wudang Taijiquan. Grandmaster Liang has been one of the most renowned Wushu masters in China. He immigrated to the United States in 1996, and currently resides in Oakland, CA. Grandmaster Liang is considered to be a pioneer in developing Chinese martial arts in the West during the past five years.

About the Author

Dr. Yang, Jwing-Ming, Ph.D. 楊俊敏博士

Dr. Yang, Jwing-Ming was born on August 11th, 1946, in Xinzhu Xian (新竹縣), Taiwan (台灣), Republic of China (中華民國). He started his Wushu (武術)(Gongfu or Kung Fu, 功夫) training at the age of fifteen under the Shaolin White Crane (Bai He, 少林白鶴) Master Cheng, Gin-Gsao (曾金灶)(1911-1976). Master Cheng originally learned Taizuquan (太祖拳) from his grandfather

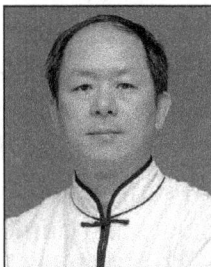
Dr. Yang, Jwing-Ming

when he was a child. When Master Cheng was fifteen years old, he started learning White Crane from Master Jin, Shao-Feng (金紹峰), and followed him for twenty-three years until Master Jin's death.

In thirteen years of study (1961-1974) under Master Cheng, Dr. Yang became an expert in the White Crane Style of Chinese martial arts, which includes both the use of barehands and of various weapons such as saber, staff, spear, trident, two short rods, and many other weapons. With the same master he also studied White Crane Qigong (氣功), Qin Na (or Chin Na, 擒拿), Tui Na (推拿) and Dian Xue massages (點穴按摩), and herbal treatment.

At the age of sixteen, Dr. Yang began the study of Yang Style Taijiquan (楊氏太極拳) under Master Kao, Tao (高濤). After learning from Master Kao, Dr. Yang continued his study and research of Taijiquan with several masters and senior practitioners such as Master Li, Mao-Ching (李茂清) and Mr. Wilson Chen (陳威伸) in Taipei (台北). Master Li learned his Taijiquan from the well-known Master Han, Ching-Tang (韓慶堂), and Mr. Chen learned his Taijiquan from Master Zhang, Xiang-San (張祥三). Dr. Yang has mastered the Taiji barehand sequence, pushing hands, the two-man fighting sequence, Taiji sword, Taiji saber, and Taiji Qigong.

When Dr. Yang was eighteen years old he entered Tamkang College (淡江學院) in Taipei Xian to study Physics. In college he began the study of traditional Shaolin Long Fist (Changquan or Chang Chuan, 少林長拳) with Master Li, Mao-Ching at the

Tamkang College Guoshu Club (淡江國術社)(1964-1968), and eventually became an assistant instructor under Master Li. In 1971 he completed his M.S. degree in Physics at the National Taiwan University (台灣大學), and then served in the Chinese Air Force from 1971 to 1972. In the service, Dr. Yang taught Physics at the Junior Academy of the Chinese Air Force (空軍幼校) while also teaching Wushu. After being honorably discharged in 1972, he returned to Tamkang College to teach Physics and resumed study under Master Li, Mao-Ching. From Master Li, Dr. Yang learned Northern Style Wushu, which includes both barehand (especially kicking) techniques and numerous weapons.

In 1974, Dr. Yang came to the United States to study Mechanical Engineering at Purdue University. At the request of a few students, Dr. Yang began to teach Gongfu (Kung Fu), which resulted in the foundation of the Purdue University Chinese Kung Fu Research Club in the spring of 1975. While at Purdue, Dr. Yang also taught college-credited courses in Taijiquan. In May of 1978 he was awarded a Ph.D. in Mechanical Engineering by Purdue.

In 1980, Dr. Yang moved to Houston to work for Texas Instruments. While in Houston he founded Yang's Shaolin Kung Fu Academy, which was eventually taken over by his disciple Mr. Jeffery Bolt after moving to Boston in 1982. Dr. Yang founded Yang's Martial Arts Academy (YMAA) in Boston on October 1, 1982.

In January of 1984 he gave up his engineering career to devote more time to research, writing, and teaching. In March of 1986 he purchased property in the Jamaica Plain area of Boston to be used as the headquarters of the new organization, Yang's Martial Arts Association. The organization has continued to expand, and, as of July 1st 1989, YMAA has become just one division of Yang's Oriental Arts Association, Inc. (YOAA, Inc.).

In summary, Dr. Yang has been involved in Chinese Wushu since 1961. During this time, he has spent thirteen years learning Shaolin White Crane (Bai He), Shaolin Long Fist (Changquan), and Taijiquan. Dr. Yang has more than thirty-two years of instructional experience: seven years in Taiwan, five years at Purdue University, two years in Houston, Texas, and eighteen years in Boston, Massachusetts.

In addition, Dr. Yang has also been invited to offer seminars around the world to share his knowledge of Chinese martial arts and Qigong. The countries he has visited include Argentina, Austria, Barbados, Belgium, Bermuda, Botswana, Canada, Chile, England, France, Germany, Holland, Hungary, Ireland, Italy, Latvia, Mexico, Poland, Portugal, Saudi Arabia, Spain, South Africa, Switzerland, and Venezuela.

Since 1986, YMAA has become an international organization, which currently includes 51 schools located in Argentina, Belgium, Canada, Chile, England, France, Holland, Hungary, Ireland, Italy, Poland, Portugal, South Africa, Spain, Venezuela and the United States. Many of Dr. Yang's books and videotapes have been translated into languages such as French, Italian, Spanish, Polish, Czech, Bulgarian, Russian, Hungarian, and Iranian.

Dr. Yang has published twenty-seven other volumes on the martial arts and Qigong:

1. *Shaolin Chin Na*; Unique Publications, Inc., 1980.
2. *Shaolin Long Fist Kung Fu*; Unique Publications, Inc., 1981.
3. *Yang Style Tai Chi Chuan*; Unique Publications, Inc., 1981.
4. *Introduction to Ancient Chinese Weapons*; Unique Publications, Inc., 1985.
5. *Qigong for Health and Martial Arts*; YMAA Publication Center, 1985.
6. *Northern Shaolin Sword*; YMAA Publication Center, 1985.
7. *Tai Chi Theory and Martial Power*; YMAA Publication Center, 1986.
8. *Tai Chi Chuan Martial Applications*; YMAA Publication Center, 1986.
9. *Analysis of Shaolin Chin Na*; YMAA Publication Center, 1987.
10. *Eight Simple Qigong Exercises for Health*; YMAA Publication Center, 1988.
11. *The Root of Chinese Qigong—The Secrets of Qigong Training*; YMAA Publication Center, 1989.

12. *Muscle/Tendon Changing and Marrow/Brain Washing Chi Kung—The Secret of Youth*; YMAA Publication Center, 1989.
13. *Hsing Yi Chuan—Theory and Applications*; YMAA Publication Center, 1990.
14. *The Essence of Taiji Qigong—Health and Martial Arts*; YMAA Publication Center, 1990.
15. *Qigong for Arthritis*; YMAA Publication Center, 1991.
16. *Chinese Qigong Massage—General Massage*; YMAA Publication Center, 1992.
17. *How to Defend Yourself*; YMAA Publication Center, 1992.
18. *Baguazhang—Emei Baguazhang*; YMAA Publication Center, 1994.
19. *Comprehensive Applications of Shaolin Chin Na—The Practical Defense of Chinese Seizing Arts*; YMAA Publication Center, 1995.
20. *Taiji Chin Na—The Seizing Art of Taijiquan*; YMAA Publication Center, 1995.
21. *The Essence of Shaolin White Crane*; YMAA Publication Center, 1996.
22. *Back Pain—Chinese Qigong for Healing and Prevention*; YMAA Publication Center, 1997.
23. *Ancient Chinese Weapons*; YMAA Publication Center, 1999.
24. *Taijiquan—Classical Yang Style*; YMAA Publication Center, 1999.
25. *Tai Chi Secrets of Ancient Masters*; YMAA Publication Center, 1999.
26. *Taiji Sword—Classical Yang Style*; YMAA Publication Center, 1999.
27. *Tai Chi Secrets of Wü & Li Styles*; YMAA Publication Center, 2001.

Dr. Yang has also published the following videotapes:

1. *Yang Style Tai Chi Chuan and Its Applications*; YMAA Publication Center, 1984.
2. *Shaolin Long Fist Kung Fu—Lien Bu Chuan and Its Applications*; YMAA Publication Center, 1985.
3. *Shaolin Long Fist Kung Fu—Gung Li Chuan and Its Applications*; YMAA Publication Center, 1986.
4. *Shaolin Chin Na*; YMAA Publication Center, 1987.
5. *Wai Dan Chi Kung — The Eight Pieces of Brocade*; YMAA Publication Center, 1987.
6. *The Essence of Tai Chi Chi Kung*; YMAA Publication Center, 1990.
7. *Qigong for Arthritis*; YMAA Publication Center, 1991.
8. *Qigong Massage—Self Massage*; YMAA Publication Center, 1992.
9. *Qigong Massage—With a Partner*; YMAA Publication Center, 1992.
10. *Defend Yourself 1—Unarmed Attack*; YMAA Publication Center, 1992.
11. *Defend Yourself 2—Knife Attack*; YMAA Publication Center, 1992.
12. *Comprehensive Applications of Shaolin Chin Na 1*; YMAA Publication Center, 1995.
13. *Comprehensive Applications of Shaolin Chin Na 2*; YMAA Publication Center, 1995.
14. *Shaolin Long Fist Kung Fu—Yi Lu Mai Fu & Er Lu Mai Fu*; YMAA Publication Center, 1995.
15. *Shaolin Long Fist Kung Fu—Shi Zi Tang*; YMAA Publication Center, 1995.
16. *Taiji Chin Na*; YMAA Publication Center, 1995.
17. *Emei Baguazhang—1; Basic Training, Qigong, Eight Palms, and Applications*; YMAA Publication Center, 1995.
18. *Emei Baguazhang—2; Swimming Body Baguazhang and Its Applications*; YMAA Publication Center, 1995.
19. *Emei Baguazhang—3; Bagua Deer Hook Sword and Its Applications*; YMAA Publication Center, 1995.

20. *Xingyiquan—12 Animal Patterns and Their Applications*; YMAA Publication Center, 1995.
21. *24 and 48 Simplified Taijiquan*; YMAA Publication Center, 1995.
22. *White Crane Hard Qigong*; YMAA Publication Center, 1997.
23. *White Crane Soft Qigong*; YMAA Publication Center, 1997.
24. *Xiao Hu Yan—Intermediate Level Long Fist Sequence*; YMAA Publication Center, 1997.
25. *Back Pain—Chinese Qigong for Healing and Prevention*; YMAA Publication Center, 1997.
26. *Scientific Foundation of Chinese Qigong*; YMAA Publication Center, 1997.
27. *Taijiquan—Classical Yang Style*; YMAA Publication Center, 1999.
28. *Taiji Sword—Classical Yang Style*; YMAA Publication Center, 1999.
29. *Chin Na in Depth—Course One*; YMAA Publication Center, 2000.
30. *Chin Na in Depth—Course Two*; YMAA Publication Center, 2000.
31. *San Cai Jian & Its Applications*; YMAA Publication Center, 2000.
32. *Kun Wu Jian & Its Applications*; YMAA Publication Center, 2000.
33. *Qi Men Jian & Its Applications*; YMAA Publication Center, 2000.
34. *Chin Na in Depth—Course Three*; YMAA Publication Center, 2001.
35. *Chin Na in Depth—Course Four*; YMAA Publication Center, 2001.
34. *Chin Na in Depth—Course Five*; YMAA Publication Center, 2001.
35. *Chin Na in Depth—Course Six*; YMAA Publication Center, 2001.
36. Twelve Routines of Tan Tui; YMAA Publication Center, 2001.

Preface

Taijiquan was first introduced to the West by Master Cheng, Man-Ching (鄭曼清) during the 1960's. The original focus of his effort was to teach a method of health and relaxation. It was only after several years that the art's effectiveness in reducing stress and maintaining health became widely known.

Since president Nixon visited mainland China in 1973 and opened the gates of China's conservative and long sealed society, Asian culture, especially Chinese culture, has attracted more and more Western people. Moreover, due to an exuberant cultural exchange, many Chinese internal and external martial arts masters have arrived in the West and shared their knowledge. Since then, Western Taijiquan society has itself opened to the realization that, in addition to Cheng, Man-Ching's Taijiquan, there are many other Taijiquan styles, all of them created and developed using the same theoretical foundation.

However, most Western Taijiquan practitioners, even today, still consider Taijiquan good for only health and relaxation. They do not recognize that Taijiquan was created as a martial art in the Daoist monastery at Wudang mountain (武當山), Hubei province (湖北省), in China. Taiji theory can be traced back nearly four thousand years, to when *Yi Jing (The Book of Changes)*(易經) was first made available. Since then, the concept of Taiji has been adopted by the Chinese people and has become one of the roots or foundations of Chinese thinking and belief. Based on this root, Taijiquan martial arts (Taijiquan or "Taiji Fist") was created. Its theory and philosophy are very profound and deep. If one only pays attention to the relaxation aspect of the movements, then one will not comprehend and feel this profound philosophic root.

Through many hundreds of years gone past, countless Chinese people have practiced Taijiquan. Many of them have reached a profound level of this feeling art. Some of them have written down their understanding and findings, and have passed them down generation by generation. Generally, only those good and correct writings, after historical filtering, will survive in Taijiquan society. Even just a couple of decades ago, these documents were considered to be the secrets of their styles. It was not until recently that they have been revealed to lay society.

Many practitioners, after comprehending these documents, have re-directed themselves into the correct path of practice and in so doing have reached a deeper feeling of the art.

I am very fortunate that I could obtain these documents and study them during my thirty-nine years of Taijiquan practice. It is from these documents that I have been able to keep my practice on the correct path. It was also these documents which have caused me to ponder and ponder all the time. Many of these documents must be read a few hundred times before it is possible to comprehend the theory and feeling.

Yang style Taijiquan was created by Yang, Lu-Shan (楊露禪) in 1799, and had become very well-known and popular by the beginning of the twentieth century. The secrets hidden in this family style were not revealed to the public until the 1990's. Although most of these documents were authored by Yang, Ban-Hou (楊班侯), a member of the second generation of Yang style Taijiquan practitioners, they are the representative writings of the style. Yang, Ban-Hou has been well known for his profound understanding of the arts and also the capability of manifesting his Taiji Jin (i.e., Taiji power) to its most efficient level. This book includes forty-nine documents written by Yang, Ban-Hou. It also includes one by Yang, Lu-Shan, the creator of Yang style Taijiquan and some important points by Yang, Chen-Fu (楊澄甫), one of the third generation of Yang style practitioners. Yang, Chen-Fu has been credited with having made Yang style Taijiquan popular since 1928.

I hope this book will help Yang style Taijiquan practitioners understand the essence of this style. I also hope that, from the study of these ancient documents, serious Taijiquan practitioners will continue to search for the deep feeling and meaning of Taijiquan and continue to pass down the art.

Acknowledgments

Thanks to Grandmaster Yang, Zhen-Duo for his calligraphy and Grandmaster Liang, Qiang-Ya for his foreword. Thanks to Erik Elsemans, Roger Whidden, Paul W. Mahoney, Carol Stephenson, Afaa M. Weaver, and Chris Hartgrove for proofing the manuscript and contributing many valuable suggestions and discussions. Special thanks to the editor, James C. O'Leary.

Introduction

In the last seven centuries, many songs and poems have been composed about Taijiquan. These have played a major role in preserving the knowledge and wisdom of the masters, although in many cases the identity of the authors and the dates of origin have been lost. Since most Chinese of previous centuries were illiterate, the key points of the art were put into poems and songs, which are easier to remember than prose, and passed down orally from teacher to student. The poems were regarded as secret and were only revealed to the general public in the twentieth century.

It is very difficult to translate these ancient Chinese writings. Because of the cultural differences, many expressions would not make sense to the Westerner if translated literally. Often, knowledge of the historical context is necessary. Furthermore, since in Chinese every sound has several possible meanings, when anyone tried to understand a poem or write it down, he had to choose from among these meanings. For this reason, many of the poems have several variations. The same problem occurs when the poems are read. Many Chinese characters have several possible meanings, so reading involves interpretation of the text even for the Chinese. Also, the meaning of many words has changed over the course of time. When you add to this the grammatical differences (generally no tenses, articles, singular or plural, or differentiation between parts of speech) you find that it is almost impossible to translate Chinese literally into English. In addition to all this, the translator must have much the same experience and understanding, as well as similar intuitive feelings as the original author, in order to convey the same meaning.

With these difficulties in mind, the author has attempted to convey as much of the original meaning of the Chinese as possible, based on his own Taijiquan experience and understanding. Although it is impossible to totally translate the original meaning, the author feels he has managed to express the majority of the important points. The translation has been made as close to the original Chinese as possible, including such things as double negatives and, sometimes, idiosyncratic sentence structure. Words that are understood but not actually written in the Chinese text have been included in parentheses. Also, some Chinese words are followed by the English in parentheses, e.g. Shen (Spirit). To further assist the reader, the author has included commentary with each poem and song.

This book includes one document from Yang, Lu-Shan (楊露禪), forty-nine documents from Yang, Ban-Hou (楊班侯), and two from Yang, Chen-Fu (楊澄甫). During the translation process, the author encountered many difficulties, especially translating Yang, Ban-Hou's documents. The author had to actually guess the meaning in a few places with an eye toward the meaning of the writing. In fact, it is very common to encounter these kinds of situations when translating ancient documents. There are a few reasons for this:

1. The different languages spoken, or the writing habits generated from geographic differences. Different areas have different slang or special terminologies.

2. Different time periods of writing and translating. Different periods have different terminologies for expressing the same thing. Therefore, the same thing may be explained through different expressions in speaking and writing.

3. Different levels of understanding and thinking in Taijiquan between the original author and the person who translates the writing.

4. Some special terminologies used only in the Yang family which outside people would not be able to understand. In order to understand these terminologies, they have to be filtered through one of the offsprings of the Yang family, or through students in their direct lineage. Outsiders can only guess. However, there are exceptions.

Even with all of the above difficulties, based on my thirty-nine years of personal Taijiquan experience, I have tried my best to translate these Yang style documents and make some commentary. Wherever the writing became vague to me, I have pointed it out in the commentary. In this case, the reader will continue searching for better possible answers and explanations about the writings in these documents.

About the Yang Family[1, 2]

Yang Style Taijiquan history starts with Yang, Lu-Shan (楊露禪) (1799-1872 A.D.)(Figure 1), also known as Fu-Kuai (福魁) or Lu-Shan (祿纏). He was born at Yong Nian Xian, Guang Ping County, Hebei Province (河北，廣平府永年縣). When he was young he went to Chen Jia Gou in Henan province (河南，陳家溝) to learn Taijiquan from Chen, Chang-Xing (陳長興). When Chen, Chang-Xing stood, he was centered and upright with no leaning or tilting, like a wooden signpost, and so people called him Mr. Tablet. At that time, there were very few students outside of the Chen family who learned from Chen, Chang-Xing. Because Yang was an outside student, he was treated unfairly, but he still stayed and persevered in his practice.

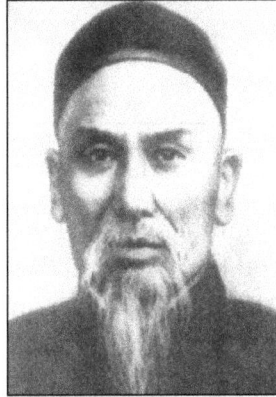

Figure 1. Yang, Lu-Shan
(1799-1872 A.D.)

One night, he was awakened by the sounds of "Hen" (哼) and "Ha" (哈) in the distance. He got up and traced the sound to an old building. Peeking through the broken wall, he saw his master Chen, Chang-Xing teaching the techniques of grasp, control, and emitting Jin (勁) in coordination with the sounds Hen and Ha. He was amazed by the techniques and from that time on, unknown to master Chen, he continued to watch this secret practice session every night. He would then return to his room to ponder and study. Because of this, his martial ability advanced rapidly. One day, Chen ordered him to spar with the other disciples. To his surprise, none of the other students could defeat him. Chen realized that Yang had great potential and after that taught him the secrets sincerely.

After Yang, Lu-Shan finished his study, he returned to his home town and taught Taijiquan for a while. People called his style Yang Quan (Yang Style, 楊拳), Mian Quan (Soft Style, 綿拳), or Hua (Neutralizing Style, 化拳), because his motions were soft and could neutralize the opponent's power. He later went to Beijing and taught

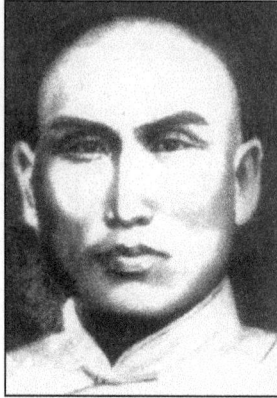

Figure 2. Yang, Ban-Hou
(1837-1892 A.D.)

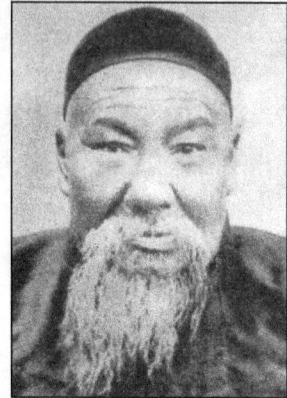

Figure 3. Yang, Jian-Hou
(1839-1917 A.D.)

a number of Qing officers. He used to carry a spear and a small bag, and travel around the country challenging well known martial artists. Although he had many fights, he never hurt anybody. Because his art was so high, nobody could defeat him. Therefore, he was called "Yang Wu Di" (楊無敵) which means "Unbeatable Yang." He had three sons, Yang, Qi (楊錡), Yang, Yu (楊鈺)(Ban-Hou, 班侯) (1837-1892 A.D.)(Figure 2), and Yang, Jian (楊鑑)(Jian-Hou, 健侯)(1839-1917 A.D.) (Figure 3). Yang, Qi died when he was young. Therefore, only the last two sons succeeded their father in the art. There are a few stories about Yang, Lu-Shan:

1. One time, when Yang was at Guang Ping (廣平), he was fighting a martial artist on the city wall. The opponent was not able to defeat him and kept retreating to the edge of the wall. Suddenly he lost his balance and was about to fall. At that moment, Yang suddenly approached him from several yards distance, grasped his foot and saved his life.

2. Yang was good at using the spear. He could pick up light objects by using his spear to adhere to the object, then tossing it up into his hand. He was also good at throwing arrows with his bare hand—he could hit the target accurately while on horse back without using a bow.

3. One rainy day, while Yang was sitting in his living room, his daughter entered from outside holding a

basin of water. When she opened the screen, she suddenly slipped on the wet step. Yang saw this and jumped up, held the screen with one hand, and caught his daughter's arm with the other. Not a drop of water splashed from the basin. From this anecdote, one can see how quick his reactions were.

4. One day, Yang was fishing at a lake. Two other martial artists were passing by and saw him. They had heard of Yang's reputation and were afraid to challenge him, so they decided to take the opportunity to push Yang into the lake and make him lose face. To their surprise, when their hands touched his back, Yang arched his back and bounced both of them into the lake.

5. When Yang was in Beijing (北京), a famous martial artist was jealous of Yang's reputation and challenged him. Yang politely refused. However, the man insisted. Yang said, "if you want to fight me, you can hit me three times first." The man was delighted and hit Yang's stomach. Yang suddenly uttered the "Ha" sound with a laugh. Before the laugh was finished, the challenger was already on the ground, bounced many yards away.

Yang's second son was Yang, Yu (楊鈺)(1837-1892 A.D.), also named Ban-Hou (班侯). People used to call him "Mr. The Second." He studied Taijiquan with his father since he was small. Even though he practiced very hard and continuously, he was still scolded and whipped by his father. He was good at free fighting. One day he was challenged by a strong martial artist. When the challenger grasped his wrist and would not let him escape, Yang, Ban-Hou suddenly used his Jin to bounce the challenger away and defeat him. He was so proud he went home and told his father. Instead of praise, his father laughed at him, because his sleeve was torn. After that, he trained harder and harder and finally became a superlative Taiji artist. Unfortunately, he didn't like to teach very much and had few students, so his art did not spread far after he died. One of his students called Wu, Quan-You (吳全佑) later taught his son Wu, Jian-Quan (鑑泉), whose art became Wu Style Taijiquan. Yang, Ban-Hou also had a son, called Zhao-Peng (兆鵬)(1875-1938 A.D.)(Figure 4), who passed on the art.

The third son of Yang, Lu-Shan was Yang, Jian (楊鑑)(1839-1917 A.D.), also named Jian-Hou (健侯) and nicknamed Jing-Hu (鏡湖). People used to call him "Mr. The Third." He also learned Taiji from his father since he was young. His personality was softer and more gentle than his brother's, and he had many followers. He taught three postures—large, medium, and small—although he specialized in the medium posture. He was also expert in

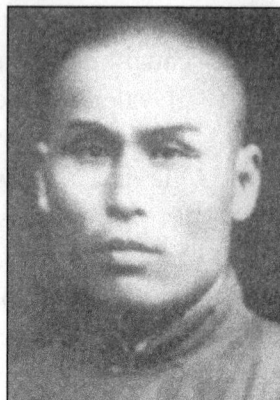

Figure 4. Yang, Zhao-Peng (1875-1938 A.D.)

using and coordinating both hard and soft power. He used to spar with his disciples who were good at sword and saber while using only a dust brush. Every time his brush touched the student's wrist, the student could not do anything but bounce out. He was also good at using the staff and spear. When his long weapon touched an opponent's weapon, the opponent could not approach him, but instead bounced away. When he emitted Jin it happened at the instant of laughing the "Ha" sound. He could also throw the small metal balls called "bullets." When he had a few balls in his hand, he could shoot three or four birds at the same time. The most impressive demonstration he performed was to put a sparrow on his hand. The bird could not fly away because when a bird takes off, it must push down first and use the reaction force to lift itself. Yang, Jian-Hou could sense the bird's power and neutralize this slight push, leaving the bird unable to take off. From this demonstration, one can understand that his Listening Jin and Neutralizing Jin must have been superb. He had three sons, Zhao-Xiong (兆熊), Zhao-Yuan (兆元), and Zhao-Qing (兆清). The second son, Zhao-Yuan died at an early age.

Yang, Jian-Hou's first son was Yang, Zhao-Xiong (兆熊)(1862-1930 A.D.), also named Meng-Xiang (夢祥) and later called Shao-Hou (少侯)(Figure 5). People used to call him "Mr. Oldest." He practiced Taijiquan since he was six years old. He had a strong and persevering personality. He was expert in free fighting and very good at using various Jins like his uncle Yang, Ban-Hou. He reached the highest level of Taiji Gongfu. Specializing in small postures, his movements were fast and sunken. Because of his personality, he didn't have too many followers. He had a son called Yang, Zhen-Sheng (振聲).

Yang, Jian-Hou's second son, Zhao-Yuan, died at a young age. The third son was Yang, Zhao-Qing (兆清)(1883-1936 A.D.), also named Cheng-Fu (澄甫)(Figure 6). People called him "Mr. The Third." His personality was mild and gentle. When he was young, he did not care for martial arts. It was not until his teens that he started studying Taiji with his father. While his father was still alive Yang, Cheng-Fu did not really understand the key secrets of Taijiquan. It was not until his

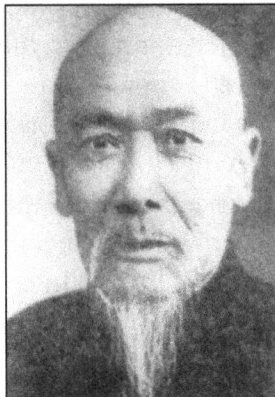

Figure 5. Yang, Shao-Hou
(1862-1930 A.D.)

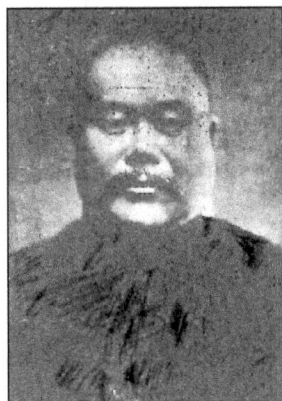

father died (1917 A.D.) that he started to practice hard. His father had helped him to build a good foundation, and after several years of practice and research he was finally able to approach the level of his father and grandfather. Because of his experiences, he modified his father's Taijiquan and specialized in large postures. This emphasis was just completely reversed from that of his father and brother. He was the first Taiji master willing to share the family secrets with the public, and because of his gentle nature he had countless students. When Nanking Central Guoshu Institute (南京中央國術館) was founded in March of 1928 A.D.[2] he was invited to be the head Taiji teacher, and his name became

Figure 6. Yang, Chen-Fu
(1883-1936 A.D.)

known throughout the country. He had four sons, Zhen-Ming (振銘), Zhen-Ji (振基), Zhen-Duo (振鐸), and Zhen-Guo (振國).

Yang Style Taijiquan can be classified into three major postures: large, medium, and small. It is also divided into three stances: high, medium, and low. Large postures were emphasized by Yang, Cheng-Fu. He taught that the stances can be either high, medium, or low, but the postures are extended, opened, and relaxed. Large postures are especially suitable for improving health. The medium posture style requires that all the forms be neither too extended nor too restricted, and the internal Jin neither totally emitted nor too conserved. Therefore, the form and Jin are smoother and more continuous than the other two styles. The medium posture style was taught by Yang, Jian-Hou. The small posture style, in which the forms are more compact and the movements light, agile, and quick, was passed down by Yang, Shao-Hou. This style specializes in the martial application of the art. In conclusion, for martial application the small postures are generally the best, although they are the most difficult, and the large posture style is best for health purposes.

1. Tai Chi Chuan: Saber, Sword, Staff, and Sparring, (太極拳，刀、劍、桿、散手合編), Chen, Yan-Lin (陳炎林), Reprinted in Taipei, Taiwan, 1943.
2. Chinese Wushu History (中國武術史), by Lin, Bo-Yuan (林伯原), Wu Zhou Publications (五洲出版社), Taipei, 1996.

Chapter 1
The Brief Summary of Taiji[3]

by Yang, Jian-Hou

太極約言 楊健侯

Light then agile, agile then mobile, mobile then variable, variable then neutralize.

輕則靈，靈則動，動則變，變則化。

Light here does not mean the body's lightness and heaviness. It means the force of attachment or the contact between you and your opponent. When you contact your opponent with light force, then can you be agile. If your contact is heavy, then there is resistance and stagnation. Consequently, your action will be slow. Once you can be agile in your movements, then the actions can be executed as you wish. When this happens, your techniques will be alive and variable. Once you can move with different variations and skills, you can neutralize any incoming attack. From this, you can see that the first step in learning Taijiquan martial applications is learning how to be light and agile. That means without muscular force.

Chapter 2
Nine Key Secrets of Taijiquan[3]

by Yang, Yu (Ban-Hou)

太極拳九訣 楊鈺（班侯）

2.1 The Secrets of Total Applications

The techniques of Taijiquan are marvelous and unlimited. It produces (the movements of) Wardoff (Peng), Rollback (Lu), Press (Ji), Push (An) and Grasp the Sparrow's Tail (Lang Que Wei). Walk (i.e., move) diagonally into Single Whip (Dan Bian) to occupy the chest area. Returning the Body and Lift the Arms (Ti Shou Shang Shi) to seal (i.e., protect) the center. Pick up the Moon from the Sea Bottom (Hai Di Lao Yue) and vary it into the Spread the Wings (Bai He Liang Chi). (Using) the picking hands (i.e., poking hand) to (attack) the soft tendons (i.e., lower part of ribs) without mercy. (The application of) Brush the Knee and Step Forward (Lou Xi Yao Bu) must be found diagonally. The variations of poking in Wave the Hands for Pi Ba (Shou Hui Pi Ba) are essential. (When) the body is closed (to the opponent), use the sideways elbow to attack. This will protect (your) center and (allow you to) use the reverse fist strike and become a hero again. (When) Step Forward for Parry and Punch (Jin Bu Ban Lan Chui), apply it to the lower ribs. As Seal as Close (Ru Feng Si Bi) is used to protect the center (of the body). The variations of the Cross Hands (Shi Zi Shou) techniques are unlimited. Embrace the Tiger to Return to the Mountain (Bao Hu Gui Shan) to complete the pluck (Cai) and split (Lie).

太極拳法妙無窮，掤攦擠按雀尾生。
斜走單鞭胸膛占，回身提手把著封。
海底撈月亮翅變，挑手軟肋不容情。
摟膝拗步斜中找，手揮琵琶穿化精。
貼身靠近橫肘上，護中反打又稱雄。
進步搬攔肋下使，如封似閉護正中。
十字手法變不盡，抱虎歸山採捌成。

This song has listed the thirty-seven postures of Yang style Taijiquan and also some of its applications. In this first section, it includes the postures of Wardoff (Peng, 掤), Rollback (Lu, 攦), Press

(Ji, 擠), Push (An, 按), Grasp the Sparrow's Tail (Lang Que Wei, 欄雀尾), Single Whip (Dan Bian, 單鞭), Lift the Arms (Ti Shou Shang Shi, 提手上勢), Pick up the Moon from the Sea Bottom (Hai Di Lao Yue, 海底撈月), Spread the Wings (Bai He Liang Chi, 白鶴亮翅), Brush the Knee and Step Forward (Lou Xi Yao Bu, 摟膝拗步), Wave the Hands for Pi Ba (Shou Hui Pi Ba, 手揮琵琶), Step Forward for Parry and Punch (Jin Bu Ban Lan Chui, 進步搬欄捶), As Seal as Close (Ru Feng Si Bi, 如封似閉), Cross Hands (Shi Zi Shou, 十字手), and Embrace the Tiger to Return to the Mountain (Bao Hu Gui Shan, 抱虎歸山). In total, there are 15 postures in this section.

Among these fifteen postures, it mentioned that when you execute the technique of Single Whip, it is used to attack the opponent's chest and the technique of Lifting the Arm is to seal and protect your body from the opponent's attack. The techniques of Pick up the Moon from the Sea Bottom and Spread the Wings can be used to attack the front lower ribs area effectively. When you apply the technique of Step Forward for Parry and Punch, you should apply it from the diagonal direction. Wave the Hands for Pi Ba can be used to bore through and neutralize an incoming attack. When the distance between you and your opponent is close, elbow strike can be used easily. Also, a reversed fist strike which follows the elbow's strike can be very powerful. Step Forward for Parry and Punch is aimed to the area of the front lower ribs. As Seal as Close is used to protect the center of the body. The technique of Cross Hands can have many variations. Finally, the technique of Embrace the Tiger to Return to the Mountain should be completed with pluck (Cai, 採) and split (Lie, 挒).

In (the technique of) Punching under the Elbow (Zhou Di Kan Chui), there is a hidden hand (for protection). Step Back Three Times and Reverse the Forearm (Dao Nian Hou) to sink the body for retreating and twisting force. The technique of Diagonal Flying (Xie Fei Shi) can be used often without being in vain. To execute Pick Up the Needle from the Sea Bottom (Hai Di Lao Zhen) the body should bow accordingly. Fan Back (Shan Tong Bei) can be achieved by pressing and supporting upward. Turn, Twist Body, and Circle the Fist (Zhuan Shen Pie Shen Chui) is a posture of dodging and neutralizing. The body should advance from sideways to accomplish this technique (Step Forward, Deflect Downward, Parry and Punch, Jin Bu Ban Lan Chui). There are techniques of sealing and seizing hidden in the wrist with reverse action. Attack the arm with the Wave Hands in the Clouds (Yun Shou) three times. Stand High to Search Out the Horse (Gao Tan Ma) is used to intercept the coming poking hand. When applying the Left and Right Separate Foot (Zuo You Fen Jiao), the hands must seal (the opponent's attack clearly). Turn and Kick with the Heel (Zhuan Shen Deng Jiao) is used to attack (the opponent's) abdomen. (When using the skill of) Stepping Forward and Strike Down with the Fist (Jin Bu Zai Chui), (you must) thrust toward the opponent directly.

肘底看捶護中手，退行三把倒轉肱。
墜身退走扳挽勁，斜飛著法用不空。
海底針要躬身就，扇通臂上托架功。
撇身捶打閃化式，橫身前進著法成。
腕中反有閉拿法，雲手三進臂上攻。
高探馬上攔手刺，左右分腳手要封。
轉身蹬腳腹上占，進步栽捶迎面沖。

Punch under the Elbow (Zhou Di Kan Chui, 肘底看捶) means beware of the fist under the elbow. The fist is to attack the center of the opponent's body. To execute the technique of Repulse the Monkey (Dao Nian Hou, 倒撵猴), you must first turn your forearm to reverse the situation. For example, when your hand has grabbed the opponent's wrist, you turn it over to lock the opponent's wrist. Therefore, you must have strong turning and twisting Jin. The are many applications of Diagonal Flying (Xie Fei Shi, 斜飛勢 ') which can be applied in different situations. When you apply the technique of Picking Up the Needle from the Sea Bottom (Hai Di Lao Zhen,

海底撈針), in order to reach the opponent's groin (i.e., needle), while your left hand is locking his elbow, you must bow slightly in order to reach his groin with your right hand. Fan Back (Shan Tong Bei, 扇通背) is used to lock the opponent's wrist and elbow and raise it upward to expose the opponent's armpit for further attack. Whenever your elbow joint is plucked, the most effective way to solve the problem is to dodge your body to the side while Circling the Fist (Zhuan Shen Pie Shen Chui, 轉身撇身捶) to attack the opponent's face. There are many possible applications in Step Forward, Deflect Downward, Parry and Punch (Jin Bu Ban Lan Chui, 進步搬攔捶). To execute this technique, you should approach the opponent from a sideways ori-

Jiquan (H-1)

Figure 7. Jiquan cavity (H-1)

entation, instead of directly facing him. In this action, there is an effective technique of seizing and sealing the cavities in the opponent's wrist area (e.g., Neiguan, 內關). When you apply the technique of Waving Hands in the Clouds (Yun Shou, 雲手), one hand is used to seize the opponent's wrist while the forearm of the other hand can lock or break the opponent's elbow. Stand High to Search Out the Horse (Gao Tan Ma, 高探馬) uses one hand to intercept and raise the incoming attack while the other hand is used to poke the armpit area (i.e., Jiquan, H-1, 極泉) (Figure 7). When the Jiquan cavity is attacked, a heart attack can be initiated. Naturally, you may also use both hands to lock the opponent's elbow upward. When you apply the technique of Separate Right Foot (Fen Jiao, 分腳), you must be sure that your opponent's arms are sealed. When the heel kick is used in Turn and Kick with the Heel (Zhuan Shen Deng Jiao, 轉身蹬腳), you are aiming at the abdominal area (i.e., Lower Dan Tian). Finally, in the technique of Stepping Forward and Striking Down with the

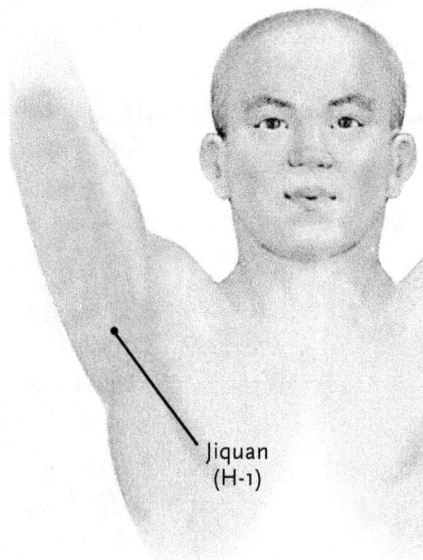

Fist (Jin Bu Zai Chui, 進步栽捶), after you have sealed the opponent's arm or kicking leg, you must approach his center quickly so you can also use your fist to strike downward to his groin.

Turn the body, use The White Snake Spits Poison (Zhuan Shen Bai She Tu Xin) to change the situation. Plucking the opponent's hand and attacking (his) two eyes. The Right Heel Kick (You Deng Jiao) is used to tread (the opponent's) soft ribs. Left and right dodging the body, the technique of Taming the Tiger (Fu Hu) is refined. The upper (hand) is to strike the ribs at the lower chest (i.e., solar plexus). The technique of Attacking the Ears with the Fists (Shuang Feng Guan Er) is effective. Left Heel Kick (Zuo Deng Jiao) is used to defend against the opponent's right heel kick. Turn the Body and Kick with the Heel (Zhuan Shen Deng Jiao) is aiming at the knee cap. The Wild Horse Parts Its Mane (Ye Ma Fen Zong) is to attack the place under the armpit. The Fair Lady Weaves with Shuttle (Yu Nu Chuan Suo) is used to seal the four corners. Use the single arm to neutralize (the incoming force) and (the other hand) attacking upward. The applications of the left and the right are all the same. Single whip to Creeps Down (i.e., The Snake Creeps Down, She Shen Xia Shi) is to follow the coming force and enter. (Then) use The Golden Rooster Stands on One Leg to occupy the advantageous position

反身白蛇吐信變，採住敵手取雙瞳。
右蹬腳上軟肋踹，左右彼身伏虎精。
上打正胸肋下用，雙風貫耳著法靈。
左蹬腳踢右蹬式，回身蹬腳膝骨迎。
野馬分鬃攻腋下，玉女穿梭四角封。
搖化單臂托手上，左右用法一般同。
單鞭下式順鋒入，金雞獨立占上風。

When you turn your body to initiate a sudden attack to the opponent positioned behind you with The White Snake Turns Its Body and Spits Poison (Zhuan Shen Bai She Tu Xin, 轉身白蛇吐信), if possible, pluck his wrist with one hand and use the other to attack his eyes. The target of the technique Kick Right with Heel (You Deng Jiao, 右蹬腳) is the lower ribs or solar plexus area. In order to execute the technique of Striking the Tiger (Da Hu, 打虎) safely, you must move your body to the opponent's sides. The attack can be to the chest or under the armpit area. Attack the Ears with the Fists (Shuang Feng Guan Er, 雙風貫耳) can be used effectively when the opponent is grabbing your chest. When the opponent is kicking at you, you can also use a kick to intercept the incoming kicks. Since the fighting range is close, normally, when a kick is used in Taijiquan, it will be low and often aimed for the knee area. When The Wild Horse Parts Its Mane (Ye Ma Fen Zong, 野馬分鬃) is used, the attack is focused on the area under the armpit. The Fair Lady Weaves with Shuttle (Yu Nu Chuan Suo, 玉女穿梭) is used to seal the four corners. One hand is used to block and raise up the opponent's incoming arm, the other is used to attack the area under the opponent's armpit. The Snake Creeps Down (She Shen Xia Shi, 蛇身下勢) is used to coil and wrap the opponent's incoming arm and then immediately follow his arm to attack him. One of the effective techniques right after this posture is The Golden Rooster Stands on One Leg (Jin Ji Du Li, 金雞獨立). Use one arm to seal the opponent's arm while using the knee to attack the opponent's groin area.

Raising up the knee to attack the vital place (i.e., groin). (When) there is an injury at the lower area by two feet, it is hard to show mercy. When Cross Leg (Shi Zi Tui) is used, the soft bone (i.e., sternum) will be broken. Before using Brushing Knee and Punching Down (Lou Xi Zhi Dang Chui), Kao (i.e., bump) is first used as a vanguard. Step Forward to the Seven Stars (Shang Bu Qi Xing) is a posture of using the hands to block. Step Back and Ride the Tiger (Tui Bu Kua Hu) is to dodge directly. Turn the Body and Sweep the Lotus

*with the Leg (Zhuan Shen Bai Lian) should be execut-
ed carefully with the protection of legs. Draw the Bow
and Shoot the Tiger (Wan Gong She Hu) is to raise up
(the opponent's attack) and to attack (his) chest. Seal
Tightly (Ru Feng Si Bi) is used to beware of the left,
look to the right, and central equilibrium. Then Close
Taiji Hands (He Taiji) to complete the postures. The
total applications of entire (Taiji), the Yi is the most
important. The body is loose, the Qi is firm, and the
spirit is condensed.*

提膝上打致命處，下傷二足難留情。
十字腿法軟骨斷，指襠捶下靠為鋒。
上步七星架手式，退步跨虎閃正中。
轉身擺蓮護腿進，彎弓射虎挑打胸。
如封似閉顧盼定，太極合手式完成。
全體大用意為主，體鬆氣固神要凝。

When the knee attacks the opponent's groin area, it can be vital
and deadly. When Cross Leg (Shi Zi Tui, 十字腿) is used, first you
trap and pluck the opponent's arms while using your leg to kick his
sternum. When the sternum is attacked, death can result. In order to
use your fist to attack the opponent's groin, you must first bump your
opponent off balance and take this opportunity to attack. Step
Forward to the Seven Stars (Shang Bu Qi Xing, 上步七星) is used to
block the opponent's attack which will offer you an opportunity to
kick him with your leg. Step Back and Ride the Tiger (Tui Bu Kua
Hu, 退步跨虎) is to step back to avoid the opponent's attack or grab.
Turn the Body and Sweep the Lotus with the Leg (Zhuan Shen Bai
Lian, 轉身擺蓮) should be executed carefully to protect the legs from
injuries and from attacks. Draw the Bow and Shoot the Tiger (Wan
Gong She Hu, 彎弓射虎) is to block the opponent's incoming attack
upward and to attack the opponent's chest. Seal Tightly (Ru Feng Si
Bi, 如封似閉) is used to protect your center. Then Close Taiji Hands
(He Taiji, 合太極) to complete the postures. To execute all of the
Taijiquan applications effectively, the Yi is most important.
Moreover, the body should be loose, the Qi should be firmed, and
the spirit must be condensed.

十
三
字
行
功
訣

2.2 Thirteen Secret Words of Practicing

The thirteen words are: Peng (Wardoff), Lu (Rollback), Ji (Press), An (Push), Cai (Pluck), Lie (Split), Zhou (Elbow), Kao (Bump), Jin (Advance), Tui (Retreat), Gu (Beware of the Left), Pan (Look to the Right), and Ding (Central Equilibrium).

十三字是：〝掤、擺、擠、按、採、挒、肘、靠、
進、退、顧、盼、定。〞

This sentence lists the name of thirteen postures.

The oral secrets are: In the Peng (i.e., wardoff) technique, both arms are roundly expanding. (Then) the movements and the calmness, the insubstantial and substantial can be used to attack (the opponent) as wished. When hands are connected (to the opponent), use Lu (i.e., rollback) to open and (immediately) use the Ji palm (i.e., press with palm) to attack. (In this case) even if the opponent wishes to return his attack (i.e., counterattack), it is hard for him to do so. When the An (i.e., push) technique is applied, (it's power) is likely to (cause) collapsing. (Use) two hands to Cai (i.e., pluck)(the opponent) do not lose it easily. (When) the coming force is fierce, (immediately) apply the Lie (i.e., split) technique. (Use) Zhou (i.e., elbow) and Kao (i.e., bump) as wish following the opponent's situation. Jin (i.e., advance), Tui (i.e., retreat), or reversed to the sideways, (I) step following the opportunity. (In this case), why should (I) be afraid that the opponent's martial art is refined. When (I) encounter the opponent and advance forward closely to strike (him), Gu (i.e., pay attention) three (out of ten)(i.e., 30 percent) to the front and Pan (i.e., beware of) seven (out of ten)(i.e., 70 percent) removed (to the right). When the opponent

advances forward closely to attack me, (I) dodge away
from the center, stabilize myself to attack sideways. (If
you) ponder and refine the meaning of the techniques
in the Taiji thirteen words, its marvelousness will grow
even more (than ever).

口訣為：
掤手兩臂要圓撐，動靜虛實任意攻。
搭手攄開擠掌使，敵欲還著熱難逞。
按手用著似傾倒，二把採住不放鬆。
來勢凶猛捌手用，肘靠隨敵任意行。
進退反側應機走，何怕敵人藝業精。
遇敵上前迫近打，顧住三前盼七星。
敵人逼近來打我，閃開正中定橫中。
太極十三字法中，精意揣摩妙更生。

Peng Jin (掤勁) is the first and the most important Jin pattern in
the Taijiquan thirteen postures. Peng Jin is constructed with both
arms round, chest sunk, and the back arced out. From the chest to
the end of the finger tips, manifest a round and expanded Qi enve-
lope. Once you have formed this Jin effectively and can apply it skillfully, you can handle any possible attack from the opponent. As soon
as you touch the opponent's arm, immediately use Lu Jin (攄勁) to
rollback and neutralize his arm to the side. This will open his chest
area for your further attack. If you can apply this effectively, it will be
very difficult for your opponent to defend himself.

When An Jin (按勁) is used, it is strong, powerful, and aggressive.
An Jin is commonly used to uproot an opponent and make him fall.
There are two places where Cai Jin (採勁) can be used effectively.
These two places are the wrist and the elbow. Once you have caught
the right opportunity and have plucked the opponent, you should not
let him get loose and get away easily. When your opponent's hand is
plucked, it will be controlled just like it is in a handcuff. However,
you should always remember that plucking is not grabbing. When
you grab, you will be tensed. When you are tensed, the Qi circulation
will be stagnant and the feeling of your hands will be slow. In addition, once you are tensed, your opponent can use the stiffness of your
body to find your center easily.

If the opponent's incoming force is very powerful, the best skill for handling the situation is to lead the incoming power to the sides by using Lie Jin (挒勁). However, if the distance between you and your opponent has become urgent, then Zhou Jin (肘勁) can be effectively applied to the situation.

When you advance or retreat, you must find and respond to the advantageous situation and timing. Otherwise, your strategic stepping action will be in vain. When an opponent advances into the short range to attack you, your mind and strategy is one third beware of the front and two thirds paying attention to retreating or moving to the sides. This means using defense as an offensive strategy. In this case, you can ease the urgent situation. However, if the opponent is approaching so aggressively that you cannot use a retreating strategy quickly, then immediately dodge away from the central line (i.e., the line between the opponent and you) and attack him from the side angle. The secrets of Taijiquan martial techniques are hidden among these thirteen words. If you can figure out their deep meaning and master the skills, then their marvelousness will be beyond what you can expect.

2.3 Thirteen Secret Words of Applications

When encountering the opponent's Peng (i.e., Wardoff), do not enter the territory (i.e., formed in his arcing arms). (When this happens), to attach and adhere (with the opponent) without separating is really difficult. To shut off the Peng must use the Cai (i.e., Pluck) and Lie (i.e., Split). When these two techniques have become real (i.e., succeeded), (the opponent will be) urgent without rescue. An (i.e., Push) can be used to firm the four sides, consequently, the corners have different variations. Once attaching with (opponent's) hands, immediately occupy the most (advantageous position) first. Lu (i.e., Rollback) and Ji (i.e., Press) two techniques should be applied when the opportunities allow. When Zhou (i.e., Elbow) and Kao (i.e., Bump) are used to attack, the heels are ahead first (i.e., techniques follow stepping). When there is an opportunity and an advantageous position, advance forward and retreat backward (to seize the opportunity). Gu (i.e., Beware of the Left) and Pan (i.e., Look to the Right) are used within one third front and two thirds rear of attention. The solid power of the entire body depends on the Yi (i.e., mind) and Ding (i.e., Central Equilibrium). (The skills of) Ting (i.e., Listening Jin) and probe (the opponent's intention)(i.e., Understanding Jin), follow and (then) neutralize are all related to the spirit and Qi. (When) seeing the (opponent's) firmness, (I) do not attack (but) gain (i.e., keep) my offensive situation (i.e., advantageous position). When is the day that the Gongfu can be accomplished is (the day) when the entire body acts as a complete unit. (If) training without following the applications of the body (i.e., postures), (even) have cultivated (i.e., trained) until the end (i.e., death) the art is (still) hard to refine.

十三字用功訣

逢手遇掤莫入盤，粘沾不離得著難。
閉掤要上採挒法，二把得實急無援。
按定四正隅方變，觸手即占先上先。
�擠二法趁機使，肘靠攻在腳跟前。
遇機得勢進退走，三前七星顧盼間。
周身實力意中定，聽探順化神氣關。
見實不上得攻手，何日功夫是體全。
操練不按體中用，修到終期藝難精。

When you encounter an opponent who is good at applying Peng Jin (掤勁)(i.e., Wardoff Jin) in combat, you must be careful not to enter the territory where the Peng Jin is manifested. This is simply because when he has manifested his Peng Jin in his posture, he is steady and firm in his central equilibrium. When you enter this Jin, you will be put into a disadvantageous situation immediately. In addition, once your opponent has mastered the skill of Peng Jin, it will be very difficult for you to attach and adhere with him. The best way of dealing with the Peng Jin is by using Cai Jin (採勁)(i.e., Pluck Jin) and Lie Jin (挒勁)(i.e., Split Jin) to lead his central equilibrium away and dissolve his Peng Jin defensive circle. If you can use these two Jins skillfully, you will have put your opponent into an urgent situation.

An Jin (按勁)(i.e., Press Down Jin) is commonly used to seal the opponent's arms down to put you into an advantageous situation for your action. Lu Jin (攦勁)(i.e., Rollback Jin) and Ji Jin (擠勁)(i.e., Squeeze or Press Jin) are often applied together and become an effective defensive-offensive technique and Jin combination. However, to make it effective, you must wait for or create the right opportunity and timing. Since Zhou Jin (肘勁)(i.e., Elbow Jin) and Kao Jin (靠勁) (i.e., Bump Jin) are short range attacking skills, when you use them you will need advancing steps to get into the short range. In addition, this advancing stepping will also create momentum for the attacks.

How you catch advantageous positions and timing relies on how effectively you can Jin (進)(i.e., Advance) and Tui (退)(i.e., Retreat). When you are stepping to set up a new strategy, you should be more defensive and pay one third of your attention to advancing, and two thirds to retreating. In addition, you must also be aware of your left (Gu, 顧) and pay attention to your right (Pan, 盼).

However, your capability for combat most importantly relies on how well you keep yourself centered and rooted both physically and mentally (Zhong Ding, 中定)(i.e., Central Equilibrium). When you are centered mentally, your mind will be calm and your judgement will be accurate and fast. When you are centered physically, you are balanced and rooted and this will give you a firm root for your spirit's upraising. When this happens, your alertness will reach a high level, which allows you to respond to any situation quickly and accurately. Your Listening Jin (i.e., skin feeling) and Neutralizing Jin can also be carried out effectively.

When you see that your opponent is firm both mentally and physically, you should not attack without being cautious. How you reach to a high level of Gongfu depends on how completely you can comprehend the thirteen postures. If you only practice, without being able to comprehend these thirteen basic Jin patterns, you will never reach a proficient level of Taijiquan in your lifetime.

八字法訣

2.4 Eight Secret Words of Techniques

(Among) three exchanges (of techniques), there are two Lu (i.e., Rollback) and one Ji (i.e., Press) or An (Push). Once (you have) attached the opponent's arms and encountered the Peng (i.e., Wardoff), (you) should not allow (the opponent to) go first. (When) there is a hardness within softness, it is impossible to break through. (If) there is no softness within hardness, then it is not really strong. To avoid the opponent's offense and defense, (you) must use Cai (i.e., Pluck) and Lie (i.e., Split). The power is (manifested) with the surprising springing spiral (force). (When) there is an advantageous situation, advance closely to the (opponent's) body and use Zhou (i.e., Elbow). (When) using Kao (i.e., Bump), the shoulders, hips, or knees are the first (place) to be used for striking.

三換二攦一擠按，搭手遇掤莫讓先。
柔裡有剛攻不破，剛中無柔不為堅。
避人攻守要採挒，力在惊彈走螺旋。
逞勢進取貼身肘，肩胯膝打靠為先。

If there are three techniques exchanged between you and your opponent, the ratio of using the techniques of Lu (攦)(i.e., Rollback) and Ji (擠)(i.e., Press) or An (按) should be two to one. This implies that defensive (i.e., Rollback) is more important than offensive (i.e., Press or Push). You should use defense as your offense, and only if the opportunity and timing are appropriate for true offense should you commit.

In combat, once you have engaged the opponent, you should immediately initiate Peng Jin (掤勁). In reality, whoever has initiated Peng Jin first will have gained the advantageous position and controlled the situation. When you manifest your Jin, within the softness, there is a hardness. In this case, your opponent will not be able to enter your center and take the advantageous position. However, if there is no softness within the hardness, then the Qi cannot circulate smoothly, the feeling will be dull, and the mind will not be calm. In this case, even if you have the hardness, this hardness will not last long.

The best techniques to defend against the opponent's attack is using pluck and split. When these two Jins are applied, a springing spiral force should be adopted. When the opportunity and timing are right, advance aggressively into the short range, and this will allow you to use elbow (i.e., Zhou, 肘) or bump (i.e., Kao, 靠) to strike. When you use the bumping technique, the shoulders, hips, thighs, and knees are the first places to be used.

虛
實
訣

2.5 The Secrets of Insubstantial and Substantial

(The success of manifesting) insubstantial, insubstantial-substantial, and substantial (strategies) is (all hidden) in the meeting (i.e., gathering or concentration) of the spirit. Insubstantial and substantial, substantial and insubstantial, the hands (are mainly used to) perform these achievements. (If) training fist (i.e., martial arts) without knowing the theory of insubstantial and substantial, (then) wasting Gongfu and (the arts) will not be completed at the end. Defense with insubstantial and attack with substantial, the tricky (keys) are in the palms. (If only) keep the center substantial without attacking, the art will be hard to refine. Insubstantial and substantial must have their reasons as the insubstantial and substantial. (If you know how to apply) insubstantial, insubstantial-substantial, and substantial, then the attack will not be in vain.

虛虛實實神會中，虛實實虛手行功。
練拳不諳虛實理，枉費功夫終無成。
虛守實發掌中竅，中實不發藝難精。
虛實自有虛實在，實實虛虛攻不空。

In a battle, you must be familiar with the strategies of insubstantial and substantial. Insubstantial means a fake action or feigned strategy, which is classified as Yin, while real action or strategy is considered as substantial, which is classified as Yang. If you are not familiar with these two strategies, your opponent can figure out your intention easily and defeat you. However, the effectiveness with which these two strategies can be executed depends on how high your spirit is. If your spirit is high, you will be in a high level of alertness and awareness. When this happens, you can exchange your strategies and respond to your opponent's actions quickly and skillfully.

In Taijiquan, almost all of the insubstantial and substantial strategies are executed from the touch of your hands. This is because once you have engaged the opponent, your hands are the first parts of your body to come into contact and communicate with your opponent. Therefore, the sensitivity of your hands (i.e., Listening Jin, 聽勁) must be high so that you can see his intention and set up your insubstantial and substantial actions. Some Taijiquan pushing hands practitioners only know how to protect themselves efficiently, and do not know how to use the insubstantial and substantial strategies to change a defensive position into an offensive one. In this case, they will not be able to defeat the opponent. In fact, insubstantial and substantial (i.e., defensive and offensive) all have their purposes and reasons. Only those who have mastered these two strategies will see skill reach a proficient level.

亂
環
訣

2.6 The Secrets of Random Ring

It is the hardest to understand the techniques of random ring. The top and the bottom follow (each other) harmoniously, its marvelousness is unlimited. Trap the enemy deeply into the random ring and (use) four ounces (to repel) a thousand pounds, the techniques are then completed. The hands and feet enter together and search for (the opportunity) in the horizontal and vertical (movements). The falling (i.e., attack) of the random ring in the palms will not be empty. If (you) wish to know what are the techniques (used) in the ring, emitting, falling, pointing (i.e., cavity press), and matching, (then) immediately successful.

亂環術法最難通，上下隨合妙無窮。
陷敵深入亂環內，四兩千斤著法成。
手腳齊進橫豎找，掌中亂環落不空。
欲知環中法何在，發落點對即成功。

When you are in a matching situation with your opponent, there are three circles of offensive and defensive domains or territories. These circles are large circle (Chang Ju, 長距)(i.e., long range), middle circle (Zhong Ju, 中距)(i.e., middle range), and short circle (Duan Ju, 短距)(i.e., short range). These circles are also called rings. In a battle, you should not stay in the same ring, which allows your opponent to set up a strategy against you easily. Your rings should be variable, random, and confusing to your opponent. Not only just the size of the rings, but also the height of defensive and offensive actions should vary as well. When this happens, you will generate more confusion for your opponent and this will allow you to execute your techniques effectively and efficiently.

Once you can generate confusion in your opponent, trapping his mind and techniques in these rings, he will be placed in a defensive and disadvantageous position. When this happens, if you know how to neutralize the opponent's attack efficiently, then surely you are in the position of winning. In order to generate confusion in the rings for your opponent, you should know how to use your hands and legs (i.e., kicks) in various directions skillfully. When this happens, once you generate an attack, it will never fail. The key to successfully executing the strategy of random rings depends on four basic skills. These are emitting (i.e., attacking), falling (i.e., plucking), pointing (i.e., cavity press), and matching (i.e., attaching and adhering).

陰
陽
訣

2.7 The Secrets of Yin and Yang

There are few people who cultivate (the theory) of Taiji's Yin and Yang. Ask for (i.e., demand) the hardness (i.e., Yang) and softness (i.e., Yin) in swallow (i.e., neutralize) and spit (i.e., attack), open (i.e., extending) and close (i.e., storing). (If) the withdrawal and release of the four sides and four corners (can be) executed as you wish, (then) why should (you) worry about the variations of the movements and calmness. (When) the production and the conquest two methods can be applied as desired, to dodge or to advance can all be found in the movements. How to apply the lightness and heaviness in the insubstantial and substantial, (the key is) do not hesitate to manifest the light in the heaviness.

太極陰陽少人修，吞吐開合問剛柔。
正隅收放任君走，動靜變化何須愁。
生剋二法隨著用，閃進全在動中求。
輕重虛實怎的是，重裡現輕勿稍留。

Though there are many people who practice Taijiquan, very few really ponder the meaning and the applications of the Taiji concept and Yin-Yang theory. Wang, Zong-Yue (王宗岳 said: "What is Taiji? It is generated from Wuji, and is a pivotal function of movements and stillness. It is the mother of Yin and Yang. When it moves, it divides. At rest, it reunites." This implies that Taiji is neither a Wuji (無極) (i.e., no extremity) state nor a Yin-Yang dividing state. Instead, Taiji is the force or the natural intention of derivation or unification. When this concept is applied into the Taijiquan practice, it clearly implies that the Taiji is the mind of the practitioner. It is your mind which directs you from the Wuji state to the Yin-Yang state and vice versa. Therefore, it is your mind that generates the Yin and Yang.

Once you have comprehended this concept, you will have seen that it is your mind which makes you change your strategies and also decides all of the actions. From the mind you can be light or heavy, insubstantial or substantial, emitting or storing, hard or soft, releasing or withdrawing, still or active, and dodging or advancing, etc. Once you have mastered these strategic actions skillfully and reached to the stage of "regulating without regulating" (不調而自調), then you will be a proficient Taijiquan master.

十
八
在
訣

2.8 The Secrets of Eighteen Dependencies

(The key to) Peng (i.e., Wardoff) is on the two arms. (The key to) Lu (i.e., Rollback) is on the palms. (The key to) Ji (i.e., Press) is on the back of hands. (The key to) An (i.e., Push) is on the waist. (The key to) Cai (i.e., Pluck) is on the ten fingers. (The key to) Lie (i.e., Split) is on the two forearms. (The key to) Zhou (i.e., Elbow) is used when bent. (The key to) Kao (i.e., Bump) is on shoulders and chest. (The key to) Jin (i.e., Advance) is on Wave Hands in Clouds. (The key to) Tui (i.e., Retreat) is on turning the forearm (i.e., Repulse the Monkey). (The key to) Gu (i.e., Bewaring) is one-third on the front. (The key to) Pan (i.e., Looking) is two-thirds on the rear. (The key to) Ding (i.e., Steadiness) is on the gaps (i.e., leisure). (The key to) Zhong (i.e., Center) is on sideways (balance). (The problem of) Zhi (i.e., Stagnation) is on double weighting. (The key to) Tong (i.e., Fluency) is on single lightness. (The key to) Xu (i.e., Insubstantial) is on defense. (The key to) Shi (i.e., Substantial) is on thrusting (forward).

掤在兩臂，攦在掌中，擠在手背，按在腰攻，採在十指，
捌在兩肱，肘在曲使，靠在肩胸，進在雲手，退在轉肱，
顧在三前，盼在七星，定在有隙，中在得橫，滯在雙重，
通在單輕，虛在當守，實在必沖。

When Peng Jin (掤勁)(i.e., Wardoff) is manifested, both arms are arced outward. Together with the chest, it forms a round Jin. Therefore, other than the round arcing arm posture, the chest should be contained and the back arced (Han Xiong Ba Bei, 含胸拔背). If you have done this, you have taken an advantageous position for your defense. When you perform Lu Jin (攦勁)(i.e., Rollback), the success of executing this technique depends on the sensitivity of your palms. If the feeling in your hands is sensitive, you can understand the opponent's incoming force clearly and lead it into emptiness. When you press forward with Ji Jin (擠勁)(i.e., Press), the power should be focused on the back of the hand. When you use the An Jin (按勁) (i.e., Push Downward or Press Downward), though the contact is on your opponent's wrist or forearm, the target is his waist area. In this case, you can seal the opponent's arm from further movement. This is one of the main goals of applying An Jin. In addition, when you apply An Jin, the pressing downward power is from the sinking of your waist area. When you are sinking, you will be rooted and the techniques can be effective.

When you apply the Cai Jin (採勁)(i.e., Pluck), the effectiveness with which you can control your opponent's joints, such as his wrist, elbow, and shoulder depends on the sensitivity and strength of your fingers. Your fingers must be strong like an eagle's claw. Once they have plucked the opponent's joints, they never lose them. However, when you apply Pluck Jin, you should not grab the opponent's joints. When you grab, you will be tensed. When this happens, the Qi is stagnant, and mutual resistance between you and your opponent will be initiated. Naturally, this will provide your opponent with a good opportunity to locate and connect to your root and destroy it. When you pluck, the control must be firm yet relaxed.

When you apply Lie Jin (挒勁)(i.e., Split or Rend), the power is manifested in the forearms. In order to generate a strong and balanced Jin, while one arm is attacking, the other is spreading in the opposite direction to balance the splitting action of the attacking arm. To use Zhou Jin (肘勁)(i.e., Elbow) either to neutralize the opponent's elbow grabbing (or plucking), or to attack such as with stroke or Qin Na (or Chin Na), the elbow must be bent. When you use Kao Jin (靠勁)(i.e., Bump), though there are many places you can generate the bumping power, the most useful and effective place is your shoulder. In addition, when you attack, the best target is on the opponent's chest area. This will enable you to bump him off balance easily.

When you advance forward, make sure you have controlled the opponent's arm and immobilized his activity. The best way of doing so is by using Cloud Hands (雲手) to lock the opponent's elbow. However, when you retreat, repel the incoming force by turning your hands upward as demonstrated in Repulse the Monkey (轉肱). In this case, the opponent's attacking arm will be repelled and led away.

When you decide to initiate an action on your left hand side (左顧)(i.e., Beware of the Left), you must pay 30 percent attention to your front to avoid the opponent's action. However, if you decide to initiate an action on your right hand side (右盼)(i.e., Look to the Right), pay 70 percent attention to the rear. It is very difficult to ascertain the actual meaning in this piece of poetry passed down by Yang, Ban-Hou.

Steadiness (定) can be obtained because of extra perceived time. In Chinese, when you have a gap in your tight schedule, it is called "Xian Xi" (閒隙) and means "leisure gap." That means in order to obtain steadiness, you must be able to remain calm and truthful to handle things easily. This allows you to have extra energy and time to establish your rooting. If you are in an urgent situation, you will not be able to spend any effort in establishing your rooting and steadiness. In order to obtain Central Equilibrium (中定)(i.e., Centeredness), you must grasp the trick of balance. Balance originates from an even lateral (sideways) sensitivity.

If there is a stagnation in applying the techniques, it is usually because of double weighting (雙重)(i.e., mutual resistance). Double weighting means when your opponent places weight (i.e., pressure or force) on you, you react with another weight or force. When this happens, mutual resistance will be generated and the execution of the techniques will be stagnant.

In order to execute the technique fluidly and smoothly, you must comprehend a single word—lightness (單輕). When you are light, you can be agile and your response to your opponent's action will be swift, fluid and without hesitation. When you are in an insubstantial situation, you should pay more attention to your defense. However, when you decide to initiate a substantial attack, the decision must be precise and the action must be fast, thrusting, and powerful. If you hesitate, your substantial attacking will not be effective.

2.9 The Secrets of Five Word Classic

五字經訣

(If) the opponent enters from sideways (i.e., my empty door), (I) dodge and extend (my arms to intercept), nothing is completely empty. Carry and neutralize the opponent's Li, file and grind (i.e., exchange the skills) to try his Gong (i.e., Gongfu). Humbly content (i.e., preserve) the force and use it conservatively. Attaching and adhering do not leave the center. Follow to enter and follow to retreat and also to yield, keep (your) mind (concentrated) and do not take it easy. Control and seal the enemy's blood vessels, twist (my arm) to bend and seal following the situation. Be soft and do not use the clumsy muscular power (i.e., Li). The Peng (i.e., Wardoff) arms must be extended roundly. (When) brush to enter, the power must be round and alive. Destroy the opponent's strength and jab his sharpness. Cover and protect (the places) where the opponent's entering (i.e., attack) are fierce especially (if he) gathers (the force) into a point and attacks (my) vital place. Drop to yield and pull to save the situation and continue (the attachment) without losing it into emptiness. (Immediately) press (i.e., Ji) him with insubstantial and substantial appearance (i.e., movements), (once you are able) to bounce (him) off (balance), then you are successful.

彼從側方入，閃展無全空，擔化對方力，搓磨試其功，
歉含力蓄使，粘沾不離宗，隨進隨退走，拘意莫放鬆，
拿閉敵血脈，扳挽順勢封，軟非用拙力，棚臂要圓撐，
摟進圓活力，摧堅戳敵鋒，掩護敵猛入，撮點致命攻，
墜走牽挽勢，繼續勿失空，擠他虛實現，攤開即成功。

When the opponent has attacked your empty door (Kong Men, 空門) from the side, you should dodge while extending your hands to intercept and attach to the opponent. This will allow you to establish contact and follow with adhering. Immediately after the attachment, you should be cautious and test your opponent's power and skill.

When you are doing this, do not manifest your power and skills completely. Be conservative and defensive. It does not matter how—you must always maintain the attachment and adherence. Whenever the opponent advances or retreats, simply follow his force and fit in with your retreating and advancing strategies. Though the body is relaxed, the mind always keeps to a high degree of alertness. Once you have an opportunity, control and seal the opponent's mobility and attack his vital area. In addition, you should become familiar with the skills of twisting and bending. These two key techniques allow one to follow the opponent's incoming force and seal it. You must also be soft instead of stiff. If you are stiff, the power manifested will be dull.

In order to execute Peng Jin (掤勁)(i.e., Wardoff) effectively, your two arms must manifest a roundly expanding force. When you brush the opponent's force and advance, the power you use must be round and alive. If you do so, you can lead and neutralize the opponent's fierce attacking force into emptiness. Once you have neutralized the opponent's attacking force, you must continue to keep your alertness and avoid the opponent's following attack. Only then can you initiate your attack safely. If you have failed in your attack, immediately yield and retreat to at least maintain balance in the situation. If the opponent takes this opportunity to attack, then step to the side to become insubstantial and use Ji Jin (擠勁)(i.e., Substantial Press Jin) to attack him. Once you are able to bump him off balance, you have succeeded in creating another opportunity for your attack.

Chapter 3
Forty Taijiquan Treatises[3,6,7]

Yang, Yu (Ban-Hou)

太極法說四十篇 楊鈺（班侯）

3.1 Eight Doors and Five Steppings

八門五步

Peng (South) Kan	Lu (West) Li	Ji (East) Dui	An (North) Zhen	Orientation Eight Doors
Cai (West-North) Xun	Lie (East-South) Qian	Zhou (East-North) Kun	Kao (West-South) Gen	Orientation Eight Doors

*The Eight Doors in orientation demonstrate the princi-
ples of the Yin and Yang's reversal (i.e., cyclical)
exchanges. Complete and then repeat from beginning,
follow the way as they are (i.e., naturally). In short,
(you) must not without knowing the four sides and four
corners (i.e., Eight Doors). Peng (i.e., Wardoff), Lu (i.e.,
Rollback), Ji (i.e., Press), and An (i.e., Push) are the
hands' (Jin patterns) of four sides and Cai (i.e., Pluck),
Lie (i.e., Split), Zhou (i.e., Elbow), and Kao (i.e.,
Bump) are the hands' (Jin patterns) of four corners. By
combining the sides and corners, the orientation of the
trigrams can be acquired. Use the body to discriminate
(i.e., distinguish clearly with) the steppings and the Yi
(i.e., wisdom mind) is within the Five Phases (i.e., steppings), (consequently) the eight directions can be supported and controlled. In the Five Phases, "advance"
corresponds to fire, "retreat" corresponds to water, "look
to the left" corresponds to wood, "beware of the right"
corresponds to metal, and central equilibrium corresponds to the central earth. "Advance" and "retreat" are
the steppings corresponding to water and fire while
"look to the left" and "beware of the right" are the steppings corresponding to metal and wood. Central earth
is used as the axis of the entire operation. The Eight
Trigrams are hidden within (the hands' movements)*

and the feet step according to the Five Phases. The hands and the steppings, eight and five, the number is thirteen. These are originated from the natural thirteen (moving) patterns. Named as Eight Doors and Five Steppings.

掤（南）	攦（西）	擠（東）	按（北）
坎	離	兌	震

採（西北）	挒（東南）	肘（東北）	靠（西南）	方位
巽	乾	坤	艮	八門

方位八門，乃為陰陽顛倒之理。周而復始，隨其所行也。
總之四正四隅，不可不知矣。夫掤、攦、擠、按是四正
之手，採、挒、肘、靠是四隅之手。合隅正之手，得門
位之卦。以身分步，五行在意，支撐八面。五行者，進
步（火），退步（水），左顧（木），右盼（金），定
之方中土也。夫進退為水火之步，顧盼為金木之步。以
中土為樞機之軸，懷藏八卦，腳跐五行，手步八五，其
數十三，出於自然十三勢也。名之曰：八門五步。

　　Taijiquan is also called "thirteen postures" (i.e., action patterns)(Shi San Shi, 十三勢) which includes eight patterns of Jin (i.e., martial power) manifestation and also five strategic stepping movements. The eight Jin patterns are used to handle the eight directions' (four sides and four corners) defensive and offensive actions, while the five steppings are used to set up the best angles for the manifestation of the eight Jin patterns. These thirteen actions are also called "eight doors and five steppings" (Ba Men Wu Bu, 八門五步). The eight doors correspond with the eight directions of the Eight Trigrams (Ba Gua, 八卦) while the five steppings correspond with the Five Phases (Wu Xing, 五行). When the eight Jin patterns coordinate with the feet's stepping harmoniously and cooperatively, the movements can be smoothly natural and effective in the martial applications of Taijiquan.

　　Among the eight Jin patterns, Peng (掤)(i.e., Wardoff), Lu (攦) (i.e., Rollback), Ji (擠)(i.e., Press), and An (按)(i.e., Push) are the four major posts that support the foundation of all Taijiquan, while the other four, Cai (採)(i.e., Pluck), Lie (挒)(i.e., Split), Zhou (肘) (i.e., Elbow), and Kao (靠)(i.e., Bump) are four minor posts adding stability and flexibility. The five steppings include: Jin Bu (進步)(i.e., advance or step forward), Tui Bu (退步)(i.e., retreat or step backward), Zuo Gu (左顧)(i.e., beware of the left), You Pan (右盼)(i.e., look to the right), and Zhong Ding (中定)(i.e., central equilibrium). Among the five steppings, central equilibrium is the most important. This is because only when you are centered and balanced can you then move swiftly and naturally. Therefore, central equilibrium is the crucial key to successful stepping.

八
門
五
步
用
功
法

3.2 The Applications of Eight Doors and Five Steppings

The Eight Trigrams and the Five Phases are the natural born endowment of humanity. (We) must first understand the original reasons (i.e., meanings) of four words: Zhi Jue Yun Dong (i.e., conscious feeling in movements). After (we) have gained the conscious feeling in movements, then are we able to (know the skill of) Understanding Jin. After (knowing the skill) of Understanding Jin, then (we) are able to reach the enlightenment automatically. However, at the beginning of practice, though (we) have the original born endowment, it is still difficult for us to grab (the keys).

八卦五行，是人生成固有之良。必先明〝知覺運動〞四字之本由。知覺運動得之後，而后方能懂勁。由懂勁後，自能接及神明。然用功之初，要知知覺運動，雖固有之良，亦甚難得之于我也。

After knowing the Eight Trigrams of Taijiquan, Peng (掤)(i.e., Wardoff), Lu (攦)(i.e., Rollback), Ji (擠)(i.e., Press), An (按)(i.e., Push), Cai (採)(i.e., Pluck), Lie (挒)(i.e., Split), Zhou (肘)(i.e., Elbow), and Kao (靠)(i.e., Bump), and also the Five Phases, Jin Bu (進步)(i.e., advance or step forward), Tui Bu (退步)(i.e., retreat or step backward), Zuo Gu (左顧)(i.e., look to the left), You Pan (右盼)(i.e., beware of the right), and Zhong Ding (中定)(i.e., central equilibrium), anyone can easily perform them. These are the natural born capabilities. However, to apply these thirteen postures in Taijiquan martial arts, the task will become very difficult. The reason for this is simply because, although anyone could shape and move in the patterns, if one were to encounter an opponent, the techniques still would not be manifested correctly and skillfully. The main reason for this is because, in order to make all thirteen action patterns work, you must first understand and practice the internal aspects of each, to understand its feeling.

Such sensing is called "Listening Jin" (Ting Jin, 聽勁). In Taijiquan sparring, feeling is the language which allows you to communicate with your opponent. The more you can feel or sense your opponent, the more readily you can understand his intention (i.e., Understanding Jin)(Dong Jin, 懂勁). Naturally, like mastering a language, it will take much time and effort to reach a high level of skill in this communication. After you have practiced for a long time, you will reach a stage where, even before your opponent emits his Jin, you can already sense it and be ready for its coming (i.e., reach enlightenment). When this happens, you have completely controlled your opponent in your hands.

Therefore, in order to make all of the Taijiquan techniques useful and effective, the most important and crucial activity is to practice Listening Jin and Understanding Jin. Without knowing these two Jins, then it does not matter how beautifully you can perform the thirteen patterns—they remain dead and cannot be alively applied into action.

In summary, this paragraph explains the importance of "conscious feeling" (Zhi Jue Yun Dong, 知覺運動) during actions. Even though we are born with this feeling, we still have to practice and train for a long time before we can reach the stage of enlightenment. Enlightenment means the stage of sensitive feeling that allows you to feel the opponent's intention even before his power to the action is initiated. In *Taijiquan Classic*, it is said: "The opponent does not know me, only I know the opponent." It is also said: "the opponent does not move, I do not move; the opponent moves slightly, I move first." This is the stage of enlightenment.

固
有
分
明
法

3.3 Natural Methods of Discrimination

When a human is just born, the eyes can see, the ears can hear, the nose can smell, the mouth can eat. The color, sound, fragrance, odors, and five flavors, are all natural sensory endowment . (His) hands being able to dance and the feet being able to step, as well as (other) capabilities of the four limbs, are all natural endowment of moving function (i.e., exercises). When (we) think of this, isn't (it) that human nature is all close with each other (since birth) but the habits are far (different) due to (various) learning (background). Therefore, (we have) lost the original born endowment. If (we) wish to return (ourselves) to the natural born endowment, it is impossible to trace back the root of movement without physical actions. It is (also) impossible to regain the root of the original consciousness (i.e., natural feeling) without intellectual scholarly study (i.e., pondering or internal cultivation). Therefore, it is from the physical exercises can (we then regain our) consciousness (i.e., feeling). From transporting (the Qi), (we are able) to regain consciousness and from movements then (we can) regain understanding (of our physical action). (If) there is no transporting (of Qi), then there is no conscious feeling, if there is no movement, then there is no understanding (i.e., learning)(of our action). When transporting (the Qi) to its maximum, then the movement is initiated. When feeling is abundant (i.e., sensitive), then (you can) understand. (However,) it is easy from movements to understanding, and it is difficult to transport (the Qi) for the (sensitive) feeling. (Therefore,) (you) should first look for the understanding of feeling and exercises within self. After (you) are able to gain (this feeling and understanding) in (your) body (i.e., yourself), then you can know the opponent. (If) you are looking for knowing the opponent first, (you) may have lost your own (feeling and understanding). (You) should not (proceed) without knowing this theory. This is how Understanding Jin can be obtained.

蓋人降生之初，目能視，耳能聽，鼻能聞，口能食。顏色聲音，香臭五味，皆天然知覺固有之良；其手舞足蹈，與四肢之能，皆天然運動固有之良。思及此，是人孰無因人性近習遠，失迷固有。要想還我固有，非乃武無以尋運動之根由，非乃文無以得知覺之本原。是乃運動而知覺也。夫運而覺，動而知，不運不覺，不動不知。運極則為動，覺盛則為知，動知者易，運覺者難。先求自己知覺運動，得之于身，自能知人。要求先知人，恐失于自己，不可不知此理也。夫而後懂勁然也。

We all have had natural capabilities of seeing, listening, smelling, tasting, etc. from our sensing organs since we were born. Moreover, we also all have the capabilities of moving our hands, and walking with our feet. All of these feeling and moving abilities were naturally born with us. But why are there such differences in feeling and movements when we grow up? Might this not be because some of us keep practicing our feelings until they have reached a high level of sensitivity? Also, might there be an effect from training of our bodies, until they can be controlled by the mind efficiently and effectively?

In Taijiquan, in order to reach a high level of Listening Jin (Ting Jin, 聽勁) and Understanding Jin (Dong Jin, 懂勁), you must practice feeling, and exercise your body until your mind, feeling, and body's action unite and coordinate with one another harmoniously. You must first start from your own feeling and learn how to put this feeling into the action. Only then should you pay attention to the feeling of the opponent. Self feeling and body action are the foundation of success in this. Only if you have first built up this foundation can you establish a high level of feeling with your opponent. When this happens, you can physically react according to this information.

In summary, this paragraph explains that feeling is the language of the mind and body's communication. From this feeling, the mind can execute its decisions into physical action. Also from this feeling, you can understand the opponent's intention and action and correspond with it precisely and swiftly. However, to reach an accurate and high level of sensitive feeling is not an easy matter. It will take anyone a great deal of time and effort to ponder the theory (i.e., internal cultivation) and train (i.e., physical manifestation) before he can reach a proficient level of Listening and Understanding Jins.

3.4 Attaching, Adhering, Connecting, and Following

What is attaching? It means to raise up and pull to a higher position. What is adhering? It means reluctant to part and entangled with (the opponent). What is connecting? It means to give up yourself without parting from (the opponent). What is following? It means when the opponent is yielding, I respond (with follow). (You) should know that without clearly understanding attaching, adhering, connecting, and following, a person's conscious feeling and movements will not be developed. (In fact), the Gongfu of attaching, adhering, connecting, and following is very refined.

粘者，提上拔高之謂也。黏者，留戀繾綣之謂也。連者，舍己無離之謂也。隨者，彼走此應之謂也。要知人之知覺運動，非明粘、黏、連、隨不可。斯粘、黏、連、隨之功夫亦甚細矣。

Attaching has two meanings. The first is to intercept the opponent's incoming attack with the attachment. The word of attaching (Zhan, 粘) is constructed from two words: rice (Mi, 米) and occupy (Zhan, 占). In ancient times, glue was made from the starch of the rice. Therefore, Zhan means to attach a paper onto something with the rice glue.

Normally when you encounter a situation, you and your opponent are at a long distance without touching each other. Once your opponent initiates an attack and you intercept and stick with his attacking arm, this is called attaching.

In Taijiquan, attaching can also be used to attach to the opponent's center and make him uprooted. This can be accomplished when your hands have already stuck onto the opponent's body. Then, you initiate an attaching Jin to connect to the opponent's center, to disturb his mind, destroy his balance, make him uprooted and float. In this case, he will be confused, and his Qi will be excited, unsteady and floating. From this, you can see that attaching can be distinguished into external attaching and internal attaching.

粘、黏、連、隨

Adhering is achieved right after you have attached with the opponent's arms or center. You adhere with his arm or his center without separating. Connecting is to keep in touch without separating from your opponent. In order to reach this goal, you must first know adhering, and only then are you able to connect. Finally, following means if your opponent yields and retreats, you continue your adhering and connecting without resisting, but through following his movements. When he advances, you also do not resist or lose adhering and connecting by retreating.

All of these four key words are crucial for Taijiquan pushing hands or sparring practice. However, these four key words are built upon the level of sensitivity of your feeling. Without sensitive feeling, you will not be in a high state of alertness and awareness, and your skills cannot be developed and executed effectively.

3.5 Butting, Deficiency, Losing Contact, and Resistance

Butting means overdone it (i.e., oversufficiency). Deficiency means not enough. Losing means separating. Resistance means (using) excessive force (to respond to the coming force). (You) must know that the defaults of these four words are originated from not knowing attaching, adhering, connecting, and following. (If you are so), then it is certain that (you) do not know (how to apply) conscious feeling in actions. (When you) just learn how to match (i.e., spar) with the opponent, (you) must not without knowing these defaults. Furthermore, (you) must not (proceed) without getting rid of these defaults. (The reasons) why it is so difficult (to learn the skills) of attaching, adhering, connecting, and following is because it is not easy to avoid the butting, deficiency, losing, and resistance.

頂者，出頭之謂也。匾者，不及之謂也。丟者，離開之謂也。抗者，太過之謂也。要知于此四字之病，不但粘、黏、連、隨，斷不明知覺運動也。初學對手，不可不知也。更不可不去此病。所難者，粘、黏、連、隨，而不許頂、匾、丟、抗是所不易矣。

Butting (Ding, 頂) means that when you execute a technique or skill, you overdo it. For example, only 20 pounds is needed to bump the opponent off balance, but instead, you use 50 pounds. When this happens, your excess force may be used by the opponent to unbalance you. Deficiency (Bian, 匾) means the action or the movement has not reached the sufficient and effective level. For example, when you pluck your opponent's right wrist and pull to your right to make him lose balance, if your pulling does not reach far enough to make the opponent lose his center, he will still be able to handle the situation by using his shoulder to bump you off balance. This is called deficiency. Losing (Diu, 丟) means to lose contact or adherence with the opponent once the attaching and connecting have been initiated. Finally, Resisting (Kang, 抗) means tensing up your body to resist the incoming force or using muscular force against the incoming force. When there is incoming force attacking you, you cannot be 100 percent relaxed and follow the opponent completely. If you do, you have led the opponent's force into your body and have allowed him to accomplish his intention. What you need is four ounces of force (i.e., slight force) leading the incoming force into emptiness in order to neutralize the situation. However, if you use any force greater than what is necessary, you will cause too much tension as you strain against the incoming force. When this happens you are resisting.

If you are committing the faults of these four words, then you will have difficulty executing the skills of attaching, adhering, connecting, and following. This also implies that your feeling (i.e., Listening Jin, 聽勁) is still at the surface level. If you are a beginner, you should remember at all times to eliminate the natural habits of butting, deficiency, losing contact, and resisting. Naturally, you must always practice the skills of attaching, adhering, connecting, and following. Only then can the sensitivity of your feeling (i.e., Understanding Jin) reach to a proficient level.

3.6 Matching without Defaults

(If) butting, deficiency, losing (contact), and resisting, (it) means losing the matching manners. Why are there any default about this? It is because if (you have) lost the attaching, adhering, connecting, and following, how are you able to gain the conscious feeling (i.e., sensitive feeling) in action? (If you) are not able to know yourself, how are you able to know the opponent? What is called the matching is do not use butting, deficiency, losing, and resisting to handle the opponent. (You) must use attaching, adhering, connecting, and following to correspond with your opponent('s actions). If (you) are able to do so, then there are no defaults of matching and the conscious feeling will be obtained naturally. (In this case, you) are able to advance into the practice of Understanding Jin (Dong Jin).

> 頂、匾、丟、抗，失於對待也。所以為之病者。既失粘、
> 黏、連、隨，何以獲知覺運動？既不知己，焉能知人？
> 所謂對待者，不以頂、匾、丟、抗相對於人也。要以粘、
> 黏、連、隨等待於人也。能如是，不但無對待之病，知
> 覺運動自然得矣。可以進於懂勁之功矣。

The four defaults of butting, deficiency, losing (contact), and resisting are the most common mistakes committed by any Taijiquan practitioner. When you commit any of these four defaults, you will put yourself in a disadvantageous situation which allows your opponent to take the opportunity to destroy your balance, center, and root. In order to avoid these four defaults, you must train the skills of attaching, adhering, connecting, and following. However, how proficiently and successfully you can execute these four skills depends on the sensitivity of your feeling. The more sensitive, the greater the alertness and awareness you will have. Once you can execute these four skills proficiently, you will be able to reach to the level of Understanding Jin (Dong Jin, 懂勁).

對
待
用
功
法
守
中
土

3.7 Keeping Central Earth in Matching Practice

Keep the Central Earth (customary name is standing on the post): When there is steadiness, then there is a root. First understand the four sides of body's advancing and retreating clearly. Then Wardoff (Peng), Rollback (Lu), Press (Ji), and Push (An) four hands (i.e., techniques) can automatically (be) manifested as wished. To gain the truth (of these four techniques), (you) must spend (a great deal) of Gongfu. When the body's shape, waist, and the crown of the head are all regulated correctly, the Yi (i.e., wisdom mind) and the Qi in attaching, adhering, connecting, and following will be uniform (i.e., smooth). Correspond (i.e., coordinate) the movements and the feeling mutually, the spirit is the sovereign and the bones and the meat (i.e., muscles) are the subjects. Clearly discriminate the seventy-two stages of maturity. Naturally, you will gain both martial (i.e., physical) and scholar (i.e., internal cultivation or understanding) capabilities.

守中土〔俗名站樁〕：定之方中有根，先明四正進退身。掤、攦、擠、按自四手，須費功夫得其真。身形腰頂皆可以 ，粘、黏、連、隨意氣均。運動知覺來相應，神是君位骨肉臣。分明火候七十二，天然乃武並乃文。

Zhong Tu (中土) means Central Earth. Among the five strategic steppings (Wu Bu, 五步) in the Thirteen Postures (Shi San Shi, 十三勢), Central Earth means the central equilibrium (Zhong Ding, 中定). To reach a high level of central equilibrium, a martial practitioner will start with fundamental stances. In order to build up a firm root in this training, traditionally he will stand in Horse Stance (Ma Bu, 馬步) on stumps or on posts situated in the ground. In this training, if you do not have good balance and a firm root, you will fall easily after a few minutes of training. Therefore, fundamental stance training is often called "Zhan Zhuang" (站樁) which means "stand on the posts."

Once you can keep the central equilibrium, then you will have good balance and root. Only then can you execute the other four steppings: advance forward (Jin Bu, 進步), retreat backward (Tui Bu, 退步), beware of the left (Zuo Gu, 左顧), and look to the right (You Pan, 右盼). Once you have mastered all of the five strategic steppings, then your eight basic Jin patterns: Wardoff (Peng, 掤), Rollback (Lu, 搌), Press (Ji, 擠), Push (An, 按), Pluck (Cai, 採), Split (Lie, 挒), Elbow (Zhou, 肘), and Bump (Kao, 靠) can be executed effectively as you wish. Naturally, the height you are able to achieve in these skills depends on how much Gongfu (i.e., energy-time or effort) you have put in.

In addition to all of the above requirements, in order to execute the crucial Taijiquan skills of attaching (Zhan, 粘), adhering (Nian, 黏), connecting (Lian, 連), and following (Sui, 隨), you must also have an upright torso, good control of your waist and an upraising spirit. When your waist is loose and the spirit is high, the mind will be clear and the Qi can enter and exit the Lower Dan Tian (Xia Dan Tian, 下丹田) easily and smoothly.

Furthermore, you must also practice the mutual correspondence of the feeling (i.e., Listening Jin)(Ting Jin, 聽勁) and the body's reactions. The spirit is the sovereign while the physical body (i.e., bones and muscles) are the subjects who obey the orders. However, the communication between the sovereign and the subjects is dependent on the feeling. Feeling is the language of the body and mind. The more sensitive feeling you can build up, the more clearly you can understand the opponent's intention (i.e., Understanding Jin)(Dong Jin, 懂勁). Naturally, you can also control your physical body to respond to the situation efficiently. At the end of this song, scholar capability means feeling or internal understanding, while martial capability means action or external movement.

Traditionally, Chinese like to use seventy-two stages of processes to represent the progress of any achievement. If you can accomplish all of the seventy-two stages of this training process, you will have reached to a profound level of martial capability and a scholarly comprehension of the art.

身形腰頂

3.8 The Body's Shape, Waist, and Crown of the Head

How can (you practice Taijiquan) without (paying attention to) the body's shape (i.e., upright torso), the waist, and the crown (i.e., head is suspended). If lacking (any) one (of these three), (you) do not have to put (more) effort in Gongfu. The study of the waist and the crown (i.e., head's suspending) can never be stopped in life time. (If) the body's shape follows my wish, I (can) extend and feel comfortable. (If you) give up this truth, what can (you) reach (in) the end? Even (if you prac- tice) ten years, you will still be confused.

身形腰頂豈可無，缺一何必費工夫。腰頂窮研生不已，
身形順我自伸舒。舍此真理終何極，十年數載亦糊塗。

In Taijiquan practice, you should always pay attention to three important things. The first is that the torso should be upright. That means the tail bone is tucked in and the body is relaxed, balanced, centered, and rooted. When the body has been regulated correctly, you will feel loose, comfortable, and natural. If you miss any one of the above criteria, then your body will be tensed.

Second, the waist must be loose. The waist is the place connect- ing the upper body and the lower body. When the waist is loose, you can build up a firm connection. This will also allow the Qi to enter and exit the Lower Dan Tian easily. In *Taijiquan Classic*, it says: "The Jin is originated from the legs, mastered by the waist and man- ifested at the fingers." From this sentence, you can see that the waist is just like the steering wheel of a car. When the wheel cannot be moved easily, the car will not move smoothly and freely. It is the same in Taijiquan—when the waist is loose, it can direct the Jin to any place desired.

Finally, in order to raise up the spirit of vitality, your head must be suspended from above. The neck is relaxed and the head is upright. When this happens, the spirit is high. When the spirit is high, the Qi can be directed efficiently. Consequently the fighting morale will also be high.

3.9 Taiji Circle

It is easy to retreat from (the Taiji) circle and hard to enter (the Taiji) circle. When retreating or advancing, do not part (from the rules) that the waist (is loose) and (the head is) suspended upward. The most difficult is to keep the earth center (i.e., torso upright, central equilibrium) without losing its (adequate) position (i.e., posture). Retreating is easy and advancing is hard, (this saying) should be studied carefully. This is the Gong (i.e., Gongfu) of moving instead of stationary. Keep the body close (to the opponent's) when advancing and retreating and also compared with his shoulders (i.e., keep the same height). (You should) be able to be move like a water mill, fast or slow (as wished). The cloud dragon and the wind tigers (i.e., action of Yin and Yang), the appearances are round and spinning. (If you) wish to apply the heavenly circle (i.e., Taiji circle), (you must) start to search now. After a long, long (time of practice), it will become natural.

退圈容易進圈難，不離腰頂後與前。所難中土不離位，
退易進難仔細研。此為動工非站定，倚身進退並比肩。
能如水磨催急緩，雲龍風虎象周旋。要用天盤從此覓，
久而久之出天然。

The circle (Quan, 圈) was commonly used to define fighting ranges for defense and offense in Chinese martial society. Long range is a circle where the distance between you and your opponent is beyond the reach of kicking or punching. This range is called "large circle" (Da Quan, 大圈). Middle range describes the distance between you and your opponent that can be reached by kicking. This is called "middle circle" (Zhong Quan, 中圈). Short range is where the distance between you and your opponent can be crossed by a hand, elbow, or shoulder's attack. This is called "small circle" (Xiao Quan, 小圈). Therefore, one of the interpretations of the circle here means the short range in which you and your opponent's hands have connected and adhered to each other. This denotes a pushing hands situation.

In Taijiquan sparring, it is easier to retreat from the small circle to the middle or large circle. However, it is much more difficult to advance from the large or middle circle into the small circle—closing range and controlling the exchange is difficult and dangerous. Once you have intercepted the incoming attack and attached to the opponent's arm(s), immediately move into the small circle. Taijiquan specializes in small circle fighting, so the attaching, adhering, connecting, and following techniques can be executed effectively. Once you have entered the small circle, you should keep the distance between you and your opponent the same. Moreover, in order to have a firm root and balance while connecting, you must stay at the same height as your opponent. Otherwise, you may lose the connection suddenly.

Another interpretation of the Taiji Circle in this poem is the Taiji Circle Sticking Hands Training (Taiji Quan Chan Shou Lian Xi, 太極圈纏手練習) in traditional Yang style Taijiquan. In this practice, the hands of two matching practitioners move following the Yin (i.e., counterclockwise) and Yang (i.e., clockwise) Taiji symbols (Figure 8), while coiling around each other. The motion is generated from the legs, directed by the waist, and manifested in the hands. At the

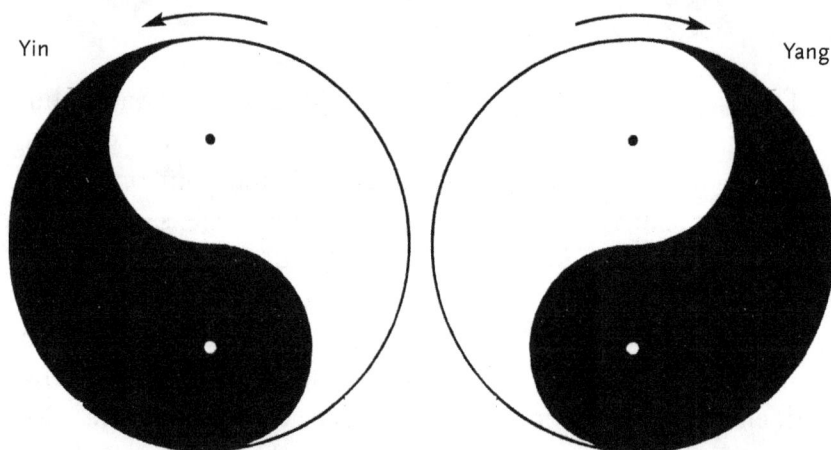

Figure 8. Yin and Yang Taiji Yin-Yang symbols

beginning, you practice along and follow the Taiji pattern, which is very similar to the Chen style's Silk Reeling Jin Coiling Training (Can Si Jin Chan Shou Lian Xi, 纏絲勁纏手練習). Later, you match with a partner while still following the Taiji pattern, coiling with each other (Figure 9). After you have mastered the skills of these Yin and Yang symbols, then you combine and intertwine the two Yin and Yang symbols. When this happens, all sorts of variations of Taiji applications can be derived. In fact, Taiji Circle training is the critical key to Yang style Taiji pushing hands and sparring.

When you are in an exchange of techniques with your opponent within the Taiji circle (i.e., sticking hands situation; short range), it is easy for you to retreat from the circle. However, if you wish to advance and enter the inner circle for an attack, you must be very careful. First, you must continue

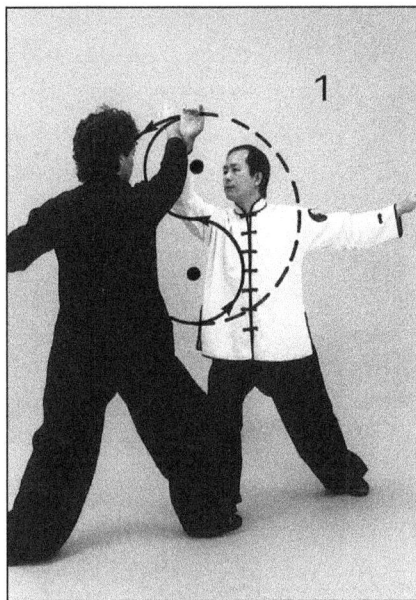

Figure 9. Taiji symbol sticking hands training with a partner

to keep your waist alive (i.e., can be moved easily) and keep your head upright (i.e., high spirit or alertness) when you advance or retreat. However, the hardest task is to keep your body upright, and maintain central equilibrium during movement. This is especially true when you advance forward. The reason for this is simply that, in order for you to step either forward or backward, you must pull your physical root. When this happens, your opponent can catch this opportunity to attack you. Normally, it is harder for your opponent to take this opportunity when you retreat. In almost any exchange with a skillful opponent, if you are advancing without knowing how to create a safe and an advantageous situation, you will be attacked immediately.

The key to being able to create an advantageous situation is to keep the distance to your opponent the same while you change angles, and to maintain the same height. If you can execute your

techniques skillfully, and are able to control the speed like the operation of a water mill (i.e., as you wish), then you can exchange your
Yin (i.e., insubstantial) and Yang (i.e., substantial) strategies effectively. Dragon and tiger have commonly been used to represent Yin
and Yang in Chinese society. In Taijiquan, this implies insubstantial
and substantial strategic actions. When the dragon appears, clouds
and rain are always coming, and when the tiger emerges, the wind
will blow (i.e., awe-inspiring). In order to understand the secrets of
the Taiji Circle, you must start to study and practice from now on.
Only if you have practiced continuously for a long period of time can
you then become proficient.

3.10 Taiji's Ceaseless Applications of Advancing and Retreating

> *Peng advances and Lu retreats are the natural theory (rules). Yin and Yang, water and fire are mutually supporting each other. First know the four hands (i.e., four sides) until (they are) real (i.e., real skillful). Only then, Cai, Lie, Zhou, and Kao can be allowed (to apply efficiently). The four corners have since derived. (The applications of) thirteen postures do not have an end. Therefore, it is called Long Fist (i.e., long sequence) which allows you to extend and condense as desired. (However, you) should never part from (the theory) of Taiji.*

掤進攦退自然理，陰陽水火既相濟。先知四手得來真，
採、挒、肘、靠方可許。四隅從此演出來，十三勢架永
無已。所以因之名長拳，任君開展與收斂，千萬不可離
太極。

Even though Wardoff Jin (Peng Jin, 掤勁) can be defensive or offensive, its goal is to set up an opportunity for advancing. Also, though Rollback Jin (Lu Jin, 攦勁) can be defensive or offensive, its goal is to create an opportunity for retreating. Only if you know the keys to advancing and retreating can you then apply the Yin and Yang strategies effectively. However, in order to make all of the Yin and Yang strategic actions effective, you must first master the skills of the four major Jin patterns: Wardoff (Peng, 掤), Rollback (Lu, 攦), Press (Ji, 擠), and Push (An, 按). Only then can the second four minor Jin patterns: Pluck (Cai, 採), Split (Lie, 挒), Elbow (Zhou, 肘), and Bump (Kao, 靠) be applied skillfully. Although Taijiquan includes only eight basic Jin patterns and five strategic stepping movements, the techniques derived from them can be so many, without limitation. Therefore, it is called Long Fist. However, even though these eight Jin patterns and five strategic steppings are the essential keys to Taijiquan, you should not forget that they are derived from Taiji theory. Therefore, you must remember this root and should never let

太極進退不已功

your thoughts or emotions be apart from it. This song points out the unlimited applications of Taiji's thirteen postures. In addition, in order to reach a proficient level of Taijiquan, you must start now and be ceaseless in your study.

3.11 Taiji's Above and Below Discriminated as the Heaven and the Earth

The above and below of the four hands (i.e., the four sides or the major Jin patterns) can be discriminated into the heaven and the earth. Pluck, split, elbow, and bump since then have had their origins. Pluck from the heaven and bump from the earth are mutually corresponding and demanding. (In this case,) how (do you) worry about that the above and the below are not supporting each other mutually. If (you) allow (the techniques) of split and elbow to be applied in a far distance (i.e., separately), (you) will have lost the (coordination of) Qian (i.e., heaven) and Kun (i.e., earth) and lament. This has explained (the theory) of circles of the heaven and the earth. When advancing, apply the techniques of split and elbow, all depend on the word of "entering."

四手上下分天地，採、挒、肘、靠由有去。採天靠地相
應求，何患上下不相濟。若使挒、肘習遠離，迷了乾坤
遺嘆息。此說亦明天地盤，進用挒、肘歸入字。

This song points out a few important ideas in Taijiquan applications. First, the four major hand Jin patterns (i.e., Wardoff, Rollback, Press, and Push) can be discriminated as heaven (i.e., Yang) and earth (i.e., Yin) depending on if the techniques are applied above or below the waist area (i.e., center). Once you understand these discriminations, then the applications of the four minor Jin patterns: Pluck (Cai, 採), Split (Lie, 挒), Elbow (Zhou, 肘), and Bump (Kao, 靠) have their roots and origins. This implies that in order to manifest the four minor Jins effectively, you must first have mastered the skills of the four major Jin patterns.

If you can comprehend the theory, then the techniques can be discriminated into Yin or Yang and applied effectively. For example, when you pluck (i.e., Cai) the opponent's elbow or wrist and lead his incoming power upward, you will have uprooted him. If you imme-diately apply bump (i.e., Kao) under his arm, you can bump him off balance easily. For another example, split (i.e., Lie) and elbow (i.e., Zhou) should be applied together. Use split to destroy the opponent's balance and use the elbow to stroke or to press him off balance. This means that when the opponent has firm balance, you must create the opportunity and take the opponent into the short range, and use split to destroy his balance. While he is trying to regain his balance, imme-diately use the elbow technique to attack him. These two techniques can be used one right after the other repeatedly.

3.12 The Achievements of Eight Words in Taiji's Human Circle

The Eight Trigrams, sides and corners, become the song of the eight words. The number thirteen, after all, is not too big. Though it is not too big, (however), if there is no balance and standard, (you will) lose (the keys of keeping) the waist (soft) and (the head) suspended upward, and sigh in lamentation. The non-stop important saying contains only two words. Carefully ponder the sovereign and subjects, the bones and the meat (i.e., muscles). If the Gongfu of internal and external are all not broken, how can (you) be wrong in sparring. When (you are) sparring with the opponent, (all reactions) are natural. To and fro (i.e., exchange techniques) repeatedly between the heaven and the earth (i.e., Yin and Yang). (We) just hope (that we are) able to give up ourselves (i.e., follow the opponent) without deep difficulty, then the top and the bottom, advance and retreat, can be executed with forever continuity.

八卦正隅八字歌，十三之數不幾何。幾何若是無平準，
丟了腰頂氣嘆哦。不斷要言只兩字，君臣骨肉細琢磨。
功夫內外均不斷，對待數兒豈錯他。對待於人出自然，
由茲往復於天地。但求舍己無深病，上下進退永連綿。

The art of Taijiquan was created based on the eight Jin (勁) patterns and five strategic stepping movements. The eight Jin patterns, called eight doors, build up a solid foundation which allows you to take care of the offensive and defensive actions from the four sides and the four corners. The five strategic steppings allow you to move forward, backward, sideways, and to maintain the center. The success of executing these thirteen actions all depends on good balance. The reason is that if there is no balance, then there is no center; if there is no center, then there is no firm root. All of this—the balance, the center, and the root—depends on the softness and mobility of the waist, and also on how upright the torso is kept.

太極人盤八字功

In addition, you must pay attention to the key words of "no broken" (不斷). This implies the Taijiquan key skills of "without resisting and without losing" (不丟不頂) and "attaching, adhering, connecting, and following" (粘黏連隨). Furthermore, when you practice Taijiquan, you must also practice both internally as well as externally. Internally means to "use the mind to lead the Qi" (以意引氣) for action. Externally means learning how to manifest the internal mind and Qi into physical action. Only then, when you encounter an opponent, will you have no doubt about how to handle the situation. Once you are in a combat situation, all of the reactions will be natural. In order to reach this level, you must practice consistently until every movement has become natural.

3.13 The Interpretation of Taiji's Essence and Applications

Li (i.e., principles and rules) is the core (i.e., main content) of the Jing (i.e., essence), Qi, and Shen (i.e., spirit); Jing, Qi, and Shen is the core of the physical body. Physical body is used for the applications of Xin (i.e., mind); Jin (i.e., martial power) and Li (i.e., muscular power) are (originated) from the applications of physical body. It is the Li (i.e., principles and rules) that the Xin and physical body have (as) their masters; It is the Yi (i.e., wisdom mind) and sincerity that the Jing, Qi, and Shen have their masters. Sincerity (i.e., truth) is the heaven Dao and those who fulfill the sincerity is the human's Dao. All of these are nothing but generated in a moment of Yi and Nian (i.e., thought hanging around you). (You) should know that by gaining the unification theory of heaven and human, then can (you) gain the Qi's circulation of the sun and moon (i.e., nature). (When there is) circulation of Qi and Yi, then the spirit of vitality will be clearly contented (i.e., demonstrated) in the Li (i.e., principles and rules) automatically. After (understanding) these, (we) can then talk about (how to apply them) in martial arts (i.e., physical actions) and scholarship (i.e., internal cultivation) and (reach) holiness and spirituality. Then (you) have) gained (the essence of the art). If (we) just focus on discussing how the martial arts are related to (our) Xin and body and apply them in the Jin and Li('s manifestation), this will have led us to the origin or the (martial) Dao. Therefore, (we) cannot just talk about the techniques only.

太極體用解

理為精氣神之體，精氣神為身之體，身為心之用，勁力
為身之用。心身有一定之主宰者，理也；精氣神有一定
之主宰者，意誠也。誠者天道，誠之者人道，俱不外意
念須臾之間。要知天人同體之理，自得日月流行之氣，
其氣意之流行，精神自隱微乎理矣。夫而後言乃武乃文，
乃聖乃神，則得矣。若特以武事論之于心身，用之于勁
力，仍歸于道之本也。故不得獨以末技云爾。

This paragraph teaches that the martial arts are our lives, and that our lives are martial arts. Through our training of martial arts, we are able to understand the natural rules and the meaning of life. Taijiquan was created in the Daoist monasteries; the final goal of this creation is to understand the meaning of the life in order to reach spiritual enlightenment. This spiritual enlightenment is the path of unification between natural spirit and human spirit (Tian Ren Tong Ti, 天人同體). The way of reaching this goal is to first understand the natural rules and principles (i.e., Li, 理). When these natural rules are applied to your life through Taijiquan, you become aware of essence (i.e., Jing, 精), energy (i.e., Qi, 氣), and spirit (i.e., Shen, 神) and the roles they play in your life. Therefore, these three treasures (i.e., San Bao, 三寶) are at the core of our being. Moreover, it is the mind that controls the body, thus, when the mind manifests itself externally, the correct body applications will result. In Taijiquan, this physical manifestation is called Jin-Li (勁力)(i.e., martial power).

It is a natural rule that the mind and body have their masters; these masters are the three treasures of essence, Qi, and spirit. However, the master of these three treasures is the truthful and sincere mind. When you are truthful and sincere, you are following the Dao of Heaven (i.e., nature) and also the Dao of a real human (Zhen Ren, 真人)(i.e., truthful human). However, all of these mental choices, right or wrong, truthful or lying, etc. can be made unconsciously, mindlessly, and can therefore cloud the mind for a long time. If we follow the Dao of nature, and are aware, truthful and sincere, then we can unify the spirit of nature and humanity (human-ness). When this happens, our lives can flow like the natural Qi cycles, as do the sun's and the moon's. Consequently, our mind, and the Qi directed by our mind, are all mastered from the spirit. This is our natural rule.

Only if you can understand the above theory, can you then reach a proficient level of martial arts practice (i.e., martial arts) and a profound comprehension of life (i.e., scholarship). In this case, you are on the right path for reaching final enlightenment. If you are only considering martial arts and how the principles relate to your body and mind for Jin's manifestation, then you have lost the most important portion of the entire training: The potential to obtain a spiritual understanding of all life (i.e., scholarship).

> *Jins are originated from tendons while Li (i.e., muscular forces) are generated from bones. If (we) discuss this by holding an object, (those who) are able to hold several hundred kilograms, this is (purely) due to the external function of skeletons, skin and hair (i.e., physical body), consequently, there is hard Li (i.e., muscular power). If (we) use the entire body to manifest the Jin, then it seems that (we) cannot even hold a few kilograms. This is due to the internal strength of the essence and Qi. Though, after being successful, if there is one who is able to marvelously manifest (his) Jin more than hard Li, then the Dao of cultivating the physical body is correct.*

勁由于筋，力由于骨。如以持物論之，有力能執數百斤，是骨節皮毛之外操也，故有硬力。如以全體之有勁，似不能持幾斤，是精氣之內壯也。雖然，若是成功後，猶有妙出于硬力者，修身體育之道有然也。

Taijiquan emphasizes the Jin's manifestation and avoids muscular Li. When Jin is manifested, the muscles are relaxed, and soft whipping power is brought from the tendons. If you use muscles, you must first have a strong bone structure to support the Li's manifestation. However, although this Li is strong and allows you to carry a heavy object, it is not the Jin in Taijiquan. This is because this muscular Li power is stagnant, shallow, and slow. Therefore, it is called "hard Li" (Ying Li, 硬力).

Taijiquan focuses on using the mind to lead the Qi to the physical body for Jin's manifestation. The body is soft, the mind is concentrated, and the Qi is strong. When this concentrated mind leads the soft whipping power to the vital cavities (i.e., vital acupuncture points), the Jin is fast, penetrating, and effectively able to shock the internal organs. Muscular Li does not take a long time to cultivate and train since it is a natural bone capability. However, it will take a long period of cultivation and practice to learn how to use the mind to lead the Qi for Jin's manifestation.

3.14 The Interpretation of Taiji's Scholarship and Martial Arts

太極文武解

The scholarship (i.e., internal understanding) is the core while the martial arts (i.e., external manifestations) are the applications. The achievement of the scholarship is demonstrated in martial arts and is the application of Jing, Qi, and Shen. It is the physical training. The achievement of the martial arts is due to the gain of the scholarship and is the manifestation of body and Xin (i.e., mind). These are the martial events. Even though, the (application of) scholarship and martial arts has its correct timing of maturity. When it is applied at the appropriate timing, it can build a (firm) foundation of physical training. When (both) the scholarship and martial arts are applied in sparring, the capability of storing and emitting (Jins) is the root of the martial matters. Therefore, when martial matter are applied scholarly, it is the soft physical exercises. (When) Jing, Qi, and Shen is manifested in the tendons' Jin, it is the martial matter manifested in martial applications, it is the hard martial arts events. It is the applications of the Xin and physical body upon the bone's force (i.e., depends on bone's structure).

文者體也，武者用也。文功在武，用于精氣神也，為之體育；武功得文，體于身心也。為之武事。夫文武猶有火候之謂，在放卷得其時中，體育之本也。文武使于對待之際，在蓄發當其可者，武事之根也。故云武事文為，柔軟體操也。精氣神之筋勁，武事武用，剛硬武事也，心身之骨力也。

When you learn anything, there are always two aspects to the learning. One is the internal theoretical understanding of the matter, and the other is the manifestation, verification, and/or the application of the theory. From theory, you gain internal comprehension. From applications, you verify and validate the usefulness of the theory. Both of these aspects mutually support each other.

In Taijiquan practice, the external manifestations (i.e., martial arts) rely on the internal understanding of the essence, Qi, and spirit. Through this understanding, and equally through the external manifestation, we are able to achieve a proficient level of physical ability. If the external function is performed without an internal understanding, then this external manifestation will be shallow. Once you acquire a reasonable understanding of the theory, then you must apply the theory into action. From the action, you gain experience. From the experience, you modify and further advance the understanding of your theory. If you can apply these internal and external aspects with correct timing continuously over time, you will soon reach a proficient level in your learning.

When this concept is applied in Taijiquan martial applications, the crucial key depends on how well you understand the theory of storing and emitting Jin internally, and also on how well you can manifest it externally. If you can only manifest the Jin externally, it is simply a health exercise. However, if you can manifest an understanding of Jin externally, then it becomes the application of both the body and the mind of a proficient Taijiquan martial artist.

If scholarship without the martial arts' readiness (i.e., support), it means there is a core with no applications. If martial arts without the companionship of scholarship, there is application without the core (i.e., understanding). It is just like a single post of wood is hard to support (the structure of a building), like a single palm will not make sound. This (theory) does not only apply in the achievements of martial arts, it applies to every thing. Scholarship is the internal Li (i.e., rule, theory, and principles) while the martial arts are the external counting (i.e., manifestation). If there is external counting (i.e., levels of achievement) without internal Li, then it must be the bravery of the blood and Qi, and (has) lost the original face (i.e., root and essence). Consequently will be defeated when encountering the opponent. However, if there is only internal Li without external counting, then just think the scholarship of peace and calmness without knowing the applications. Then when there is a battle, will die just a slight error. If (we wish) to apply the self (understanding) to the opponent, how can we not understand the interpretation of the scholarship and martial two words?

文無武之預備，為之有體無用；武無文之侶伴，為之有用無體。如獨木難支，孤掌不響，不惟體育武事之功，事事皆如此理也。文者內理也，武者外數也，有外數無內理，必為血氣之勇，失于本來面目，欺敵必敗爾；有內理，無外數，徒思安靜之學，未知用的，采戰差微則亡耳。自用于人，文武二字之解豈可不解哉？

From the above discussion, it should be clear that without physical manifestation, any internal scholarly understanding is useless. However, without an internal theoretical understanding, any external manifestation will not possess the essence and foundation. It is just like a single post which cannot by itself support a building, or a single palm that cannot make a noise. Those who know only external manifestation without knowing the internal theory can make only a proud manifestation of the blood and Qi physically. There is no internal cultivation of calmness and wisdom. In this case, you will not be able to understand the opponent and adopt the appropriate timing and opportunity for your strategic action. Conversely, if you know only internal cultivation without knowing how to apply it into physical action and application, then you will surely lose the battle. In order to achieve victory, you must understand both the opponent and yourself. This can only be done if you cultivate an internal understanding, and learn how to analyze the situation, and also know how to apply your understanding into action efficiently. You should know that the internal understanding is Yin while the external manifestation is Yang, for any study or learning.

太
極
懂
勁
解

3.15 The Interpretation of Taiji's Understanding Jin

(If) we have comprehended our Understanding Jin and reached the (level of) spiritual enlightenment, it means the scholarship (i.e., internal understanding and the sensitivity of feeling) has been accomplished and can be applied to the battle. There are seventy-two Yin (status) in a human body all the times. If Yang is able to gain Yin, the water and fire will have supported each other, Qian (i.e., heaven) and Kun (i.e., earth) will interact each other harmoniously. Consequently, life and human nature can be protected. (If) we are able to understand the opponent's Jin, then during looking and listening, encountering the variations, will obtain the marvelousness of the curve and sincerity (i.e., straight). (If) the body's shape (i.e., external action) can be clearly manifested without being tired (i.e., without effort), it is due to the sensitive feeling of the exercises. When (we) have reached this stage, (we) are able to apply (the skills) appropriately without necessity of using the Xin (i.e., mind).

自己懂勁，接及神明，為之文成而後采戰。身中之陰，
七十有二，無時不然，陽得其陰，水火既濟，乾坤交泰，
性命葆真矣。于人懂勁，視聽之際，遇而變化，自得曲
誠之妙，形著明于不勞，運動覺知也。功至此，可為攸
往咸宜，無須有心之運用耳。

The final goal of Taijiquan practice is to reach the stage of "regulating without regulating." For example, when you just start learning how to drive, your mind is in the steering wheel, brake, clutch, accelerator, etc. Therefore, you are regulating the driving, and this means you are driving with your mind focused tightly on driving. However, after you have driven for a long period of time, you can drive the car without too much tense attention, instead driving naturally and automatically. It can then be said that you are driving without driving. This is the stage of "regulating without regulating."

It is the same in Taijiquan practice. As a product of a long period of correct practice in listening, understanding, attaching, adhering, connecting, and following, you will have reached a stage of "regulating without regulating." When this happens, you can apply your skills and react to any action naturally and automatically. This is the stage approaching enlightenment. Once you have reached this stage, the body's Yin (i.e., Kun, 坤) and Yang (i.e.,Qian, 乾) will harmoniously and naturally interact with each other. This is the way of maintaining health and longevity. Moreover, when you have reached this stage, you can understand the opponent's intention and Jin, and react accordingly without any effort. This is the stage of natural reaction which is not originated from the mind.

八五十三勢長拳解

3.16 The Interpretation of the Eight Doors and Five Gates—Thirteen Postures Long Fist

When you train, after completing and become proficient in each pattern and each posture, then combine them and become long, incessantly without broken, complete and again repeat, therefore, it is named "Long Fist." (You) must not have definite postures (i.e., patterns), it is to be feared that, after practicing for a long time, it becomes the slippery fist (i.e., slippery routine). It is also to be feared that it gradually derives into hard fist (i.e., dead art). (You) must not lose its softness, the repeat movements of the entire body (i.e., continuity), and the foundation of the spirit of vitality, Yi, and Qi. After practicing them for a long time, (you) will comprehend them automatically and act as (you) wish. (Consequently,) whichever hardness cannot be destroyed. When (you are) sparring with an opponent, the four hands (techniques)(i.e., Peng, Lu, Ji, and An) must (always) be the first. These are originated from the eight doors and five steppings. Standing with these four hands, grinding (i.e., turning and coiling) with these four hands, advance and retreat with these four hands, keep the central equilibrium with these four hands, up and down with these four hands, harmonize the three powers (i.e., heaven, human, and earth) with these four hands. Start from the low level of long fist four hands, open and extend widely. After train until they have reached a stage of becoming compact and tight, bend and extend freely as wished, then (you) have ascended to the middle and top levels of skills.

自己用功，一勢一式，用成之後，合之為長，淘淘不斷，
周而復始，所以名長拳也。萬不得有一定架子，恐日久
入于滑拳也，又恐入于硬拳也。決不可失其綿軟，周身
往復，精神意氣之本，用久自然貫通，無往不至，何堅
不摧也。與人對待，四手當先，亦自八門五步而來。站
四手，四手碾磨，進退四手，中四手，上下四手，三才
四手，由下乘長拳四手起，大開大展，煉至緊湊伸屈自
由之功，則升之中上成矣。

When you practice Taijiquan, you should always first pay attention to each posture and each movement until you feel comfortable and natural. Only then, when you combine them into a long sequence, can the performance be as fluid and smooth as river water, flowing without breaking. After the entire sequence is completed, repeat it again from the beginning. It is from this repeating effort that the Taijiquan artist can become proficient. When you practice, your mind must be flexible. Taijiquan is not a dead art. It is the art manifested externally from internal feeling. If you lose this feeling, it will just become a rote, mechanical drill, and you will have lost the internal, self-cultivating feeling. Moreover, if you let it become a routine, it can make your body stiff and become a stubborn, stagnating art.

Therefore, when you practice the Taijiquan sequence, you must always first establish the internal self-sensing, or feeling. Feeling is the language of the body and the mind. From feeling, you can make the body soft from the inside out. You should always reach to the spirit (i.e., Shen, 神), the Yi (意)(i.e., wisdom mind), and the Qi. With these three things as a foundation, you will soon be able to perform your Taijiquan artfully, as you wish. Consequently, the Jin (勁) can be manifested powerfully and can defeat your opponent easily.

However, you must also remember one more important thing. When you are fighting, it does not matter what situation you are in, you should always be able to use the four hands (i.e., four skills) skillfully. These four hands are: Wardoff (i.e., Peng, 掤), Rollback (i.e., Lu, 擺), Press (i.e., Ji, 擠), and Push (i.e., An, 按). These four important Jin patterns originate from the Eight Doors (i.e., Ba Men, 八門) and the Five Steppings (i.e., Wu Bu, 五步). If you can execute these four hands proficiently in any situation such as standing, coiling, advancing, retreating, central equilibrium, up and down, etc., then have you grasped the vital key to achieve a high level in Taijiquan practice. At the beginning, your practice postures should be big, and the defensive circle should be large. However, once you have reached a proficient level, the postures should become smaller, and the defensive circle will also become more compact. To do this effectively is a high level of achievement in Taijiquan.

3.17 The Interpretation of the Reversal of Taiji's Yin and Yang

Yang symbolizes Qian (in the trigrams), heaven, sun, fire, Li (in the trigrams), releasing, exiting, emitting, confronting, opening, subject, flesh, application, Qi, physical body, martial (i.e., activities to build up the physical life), square, exhalation, upward, advancing, and corners; Yin symbolizes Kun (in the trigrams), earth, moon, water, Kan (in the trigrams), rolling, entering, storing, relating, unifying, ruler, bones, core, rules, Xin (i.e., mind), scholarly (study)(i.e., to cultivate the human nature), round, inhalation, downward, retreating, and sides. The theory of reversal (of Yin and Yang) can be clearly explained in detail by "water-fire." It is just like the flame of the fire is upward while the water is flowing downward. If (we) are able to keep the fire underneath the water, then the situation has been reversed. However, if (we) do not know the method, then this goal cannot be achieved. For example, if (we) put the water in the cauldron and placed it on the fire, then the water can be heated up from the fire underneath. In this case, the water cannot flow downward and the flame cannot be upward due to the separation of the cauldron. Therefore, there is a control which prevents the flame from going upward ceaselessly without limitation and water flowing downward continuously without stop. This is what is called the water and fire are supporting each other and is the theory of (Yin-Yang) reversal. If (we) allow the flame (to) go upward and water (to) flow downward without control, then the water and the fire cannot be coexisting and supporting each other, which results in the separation of the fire and water (i.e., cannot exist together). Therefore, it is said, when they are separated, there are two and when they are unified, they are one. Thus, one is two and two is one. In summary, it is from this rule, the Three (powers), heaven, earth, and human are derived.

太極陰陽顛倒解

陽乾、天、日、火、離、放、出、發、對、開、臣、肉、
用、氣、身、武〔立命〕、方、呼、上、進、隅；陰坤、
地、月、水、坎、卷、入、蓄、待、合、君、骨、體、
理、心、文〔盡性〕、圓、吸、下、退、正。蓋顛倒之
理，〝水火〞二字詳之則可明。如火炎上，水潤下者，
若能使火在下而用水在上，則為顛倒。然非有法治之，
則不得矣。譬如水入鼎內，而置火之上，鼎中之水，得
火以然之，不但水不能下潤，藉火氣水必有溫時，火雖
炎上，得鼎以隔之，是為有極之地，不使炎上之火無止
息，亦不使潤下之水永滲漏，此所謂水火既濟之理也，
顛倒之理也。若使任其火炎上，水潤下，必至水火必分
為二，則為水火未濟也。故云分而為二，合之為一之理
也。故云一而二，二而一，總斯理為三，天、地、人也。

Through the governing of Taiji (i.e., Dao), the Yin and Yang two poles are derived from Wuji (無極)(i.e., no extremity). Also through the governing of Taiji, the Yin and Yang can be reunited into Wuji. However, in order to have harmonious interaction of Yin and Yang, Yin and Yang must be balanced with each other. From this balance, we are able to return to the Wuji state.

You should understand that Yin and Yang are not Kan (坎) and Li (離). Kan and Li or Water and Fire are the methods (i.e., actions) which are able to influence the balance of Yin and Yang (i.e., status). Therefore, Yin and Yang are the results of Kan and Li or Water and Fire. In Taijiquan practice, if you can apply the Yin-Yang, Kan-Li theory into your practice, then your comprehension of Taijiquan will be profound. When this internal comprehension is manifested externally, your Taijiquan will be proficient. For example, Yang is related to Qian, heaven, sun, fire, Li, releasing, exiting, emitting, confronting, opening, subject, flesh, application, Qi, the physical body, martial actions, square, exhalation, upward, advancing, and corners; Yin is associated with Kun, the earth, the moon, water, Kan, rolling, entering, storing, relating, unifying, ruler, bones, core, rules, Xin, scholarly study, roundness, inhalation, downward, retreating, and four sides.

In Taijiquan, once you can understand the Yin-Yang and Kan-Li concepts, then you must learn how to apply them into all action so Yin and Yang can coexist at the same time, balancing and harmonizing each other. Where there is Yin, there also is Yang and vice versa. When this happens, Yin and Yang can be reversed anytime desired. When this happens, insubstantial can be substantial or insubstantial, and substantial can also be substantial and insubstantial. This will make your strategic action alive and exchangeable. However, if you do not comprehend the theory of Yin-Yang and Kan-Li clearly, then you will not be able to reach this goal, and your tactics and actions will not be effective.

(If you) understand this reversal theory of Yin and Yang, then we can talk about Dao. If (we) understand that (we) can never separate ourselves from Dao, then we can talk about humanity. If (we) are able to use the humanity to develop the Dao and knowing that Dao is not far from us, then (we) are able to discuss how (human) can be coexisting with the heaven and the earth. The heaven is above, the earth is below, and the human is between. If (we) are able to refer to the heaven('s laws) and observe the earth('s rules), harmonize with the brightness of the sun and the moon (i.e., timing), endure with the Five Sacred Mountains and Four Great Rivers, act together with the Four Seasons, wither and flourish with the grass and woods, comprehend the good and the bad destinies of the ghosts and deities, and know the prosperity and adversity of human affairs, then (we) are able to conclude that Qian and Kun are a big heaven and earth (i.e., macrocosm) while a human is a small heaven and earth (i.e., microcosm). Therefore, in terms of human's body and mind, if (we) are able to study the abilities of heaven and earth, then (we) are capable of understanding the innate wisdom and abilities. If (we) wish not to lose our inherent capabilities, (we must) cultivate the awe-inspiring and righteous Qi without harming it, then are (we) able to last forever (i.e., longevity). What is meant that the human body is a small heaven and earth (i.e., microcosm), implies that the heaven is the intrinsic human nature while the earth is the human physical life. The core of

a human is its insubstantial spirituality. If (we) do not understand this, how can (we) be coexisting with the heaven and the earth as Three Powers. If (we) are not able to fulfill (our) intrinsic human nature and establish a healthy life, how can (we) reach the final goal of spiritual cultivation (i.e., enlightenment)?

明此陰陽顛倒之理，則可與言道；知道不可臾離，則可
與言人；能以人弘道，知道不遠人，則可與言天地同體。
上天下地，人在其中矣。苟能參天察地，與日月合其明，
與五岳四瀆畢朽，與四時之錯行，與草木並枯榮，明鬼
神之吉凶，知人事之興衰，則可言乾坤為一大天地，人
為一小天地也。夫如人之身心，致知格物于天地之知能，
則可言人之良知良能。若思不失固有其功用，浩然正氣，
直養無害，悠久無疆矣。所謂人身生成一小天地者，天
也性也，地也命也，人也虛靈也，神也，若不明之者，
烏能配天、地為三乎？然非盡性立命、窮神達化之功，
胡為乎來哉？

We are part of nature, and therefore always follow the natural influence of Yin and Yang. In order to understand ourselves, we must first understand the natural cycles and timing of Yin and Yang. Once we have comprehended these natural cycles, we can then apply them into our body. When this happens, we can harmonize humanity with the heavens and the earth, and coexist as Three Powers (San Cai, 三才). The Five Sacred Mountains are: Song Shan (嵩山), Heng Shan (衡山), Heng Shan (恆山), Tai Shan (泰山), and Hua Shan (華山). The Four Great Rivers include: Chang Jiang (i.e., Yangtze River)(長江), Huang He (i.e., Yellow River)(黃河), Huai He (淮河), and Ji He (濟河).

3.18 The Interpretation of Taiji in the Human Life

In an entire human body, the mind (i.e., Xin) is the master of the whole body. This master is Taiji (i.e., Grand Ultimate). Two eyes are sun and moon and are the Two Poles. The head symbolizes the heaven, the feet symbolize the earth, and humanity concealed in Renzhong and Zhongwan, all together are Three Powers. Four limbs are Four Phases. Kidney-water, heart-fire, liver-wood, lung-metal, spleen-earth all belong to Yin; bladder-water, small intestine-fire, gall bladder-wood, large intestine-metal, stomach-earth all belong to Yang. These are internal aspects (of a human life). Head-fire, Dihe-Chengjiang-water, left ear-metal and right ear-wood which correspond to two Mingmen (i.e., kidneys), these are external aspects (of a human life). The spirit is originated from Xin (i.e., heart), the eyes are the sprouts of the Xin; the (original) essence is produced from the kidneys, the brain and the kidneys are the root of the essence; Qi is issued from the lungs, and the gall bladder Qi is the origin of the lungs. When the eyes' vision and thinking can be clear, the Xin will be touched and the spirit will be moved smoothly; listening makes the thinking wise, so the brain can be touched and the kidneys can be slippery (i.e., Qi is smooth). The nose's smelling of fragrance and odors and the mouth's breathing in and out, water-salty, wood-sour, earth-sweet, fire-bitter, metal-hot (taste), together with the voice in speaking, wood-bright, fire-scorched, metal-moist, earth-dusty, water-drifting, also the nose's breathing and mouth's tasting, all are due to Qi's to and fro, (they are) the gates of the lungs and (associated with) the liver and gall bladder's wind (Xun) and thunder (Zhen), (consequently), uttered as sounds and entering and exiting as the five flavors. This implies using the six unifications of the mouth, eyes, nose, tongue, spirit, and Yi (i.e., mind) to break (i.e.,

人生太極解

conquest) six desires. This belongs to the internal aspect. (We) should also make the hands, feet, shoulders, knees, elbows, and hips unified as six unifications so as to straighten out the six Daos. This belongs to the external aspect. Eyes, ears, nose, mouth, anus, urethra, and navel are the seven external orifices; happiness, anger, worry, longing (for) sorrow, fear, and shock are the seven internal emotions. All emotions are originated from Xin (i.e., mind which is related to heart). Happiness-heart, anger-liver, worry-spleen, sorrow-lungs, fear-kidneys, shock-gall bladder, longing (for)-small intestines, apprehension-bladder melancholy-stomach, anxiety-large intestine. These are internal aspects.

人之周身，心為一身之主宰。主宰，太極也。二目為日月，即兩儀也。頭象天，足象地，人中之人及中腕，合之為三才也。四肢，四象也。腎水，心火，肝木，肺金，脾土，皆屬陰；膀胱水，小腸火，膽木，大腸金，胃土，皆陽也。茲為內也。顱丁火，地閣承漿水，左耳金，右耳木，兩命門也。茲為外也。神出于心，眼目為心之苗；精出于腎，腦腎為精之本；氣出于肺，膽氣為肺之原。視思明，心動神流也；聽思聰，腦動腎滑也。鼻之嗅香臭，口之呼吸出入，水咸、木酸、土甜、火苦、金辣、及言語聲音，木亮、火焦、金潤、土堨、水漂、鼻息口呼吸之味皆氣之往來，肺之門戶，肝膽巽震之風雷，發之聲音，出入五味。此言口、目、鼻、舌、神、意、使之六合、以破六欲也，此內也；手、足、肩、膝、肘、胯，亦使六合，以正六道也，此外也。眼、耳、鼻、口、大小便、肚臍，外七竅也；喜、怒、憂、思、悲、恐、驚，內七情也。七情皆以心為主，喜心、怒肝、憂脾、悲肺、恐腎、驚膽、思小腸、怕膀胱、愁胃、慮大腸，此內也。

This paragraph explains the association of the internal feeling and the external organs and their manifestations. In the human body, the mind is the master of the entire being that makes decisions. As previously explained, the mind is Taiji (i.e., the Dao) when the concept of Taiji itself is applied to human thinking and actions. We have five sensing organs—the eyes, nose, ears, tongue (i.e., mouth), and skin which enable the collection of information from outside of our body, bringing it to our brains to facilitate decisions. In addition, when our mind obtains such information, seven different emotions and six desires are generated. The seven emotions which are associated with the seven internal organs are: happiness-heart, anger-liver, worry-spleen, sorrow-lungs, fear-kidneys, shock-gall bladder, longing (for)-small intestines, apprehension-bladder, melancholy-stomach, anxiety-large intestine. The six desires are those which originate in the six roots: the eyes, ears, nose, tongue, body, and mind. It is from these seven emotions and six desires that our mind is confused, disturbed, and scattered. From practicing Taijiquan, we learn how to harmonize and regulate our emotions and desires, and consequently bring our minds to a peaceful, calm, and harmonious state. Therefore, we must understand ourselves and our relation to nature internally, and also learn how to manifest the cultivation of our internal mind into external physical actions. From this training, heaven, human, and earth can be unified, and our natural beings can be cultivated. Renzhong (人中)(Gv-26) is an acupuncture cavity under the nose, while the Zhongwan (中脘)(Co-12) cavity is located at the solar plexus area (Figure 10). Dihe (地合)(M-HN-19) and Chengjiang (承漿)(Co-24) are located on the face (Figure 11).

Li (in the Eight Trigrams) corresponds to the south, Wu (in the Terrestrial, i.e., 11 A.M.–1 P.M.), fire, and heart primary Qi channel. Kan (in the Eight Trigrams) corresponds to the north, Zi (in the Terrestrial, i.e., 11 P.M.–1 A.M.), water, and kidney primary Qi channel. Zhen (in the Eight Trigrams) corresponds to the east, Mao (in the Terrestrial, i.e., 5-7 A.M.), fire, and heart primary Qi channel. Dui (in the Eight Trigrams) corresponds to the west, Qiu (in the Terrestrial, i.e., 5-7 P.M.), metal, and lung primary Qi channel. Qian (in the Eight Trigrams) corresponds to the west-north, metal, large intestine primary Qi channel, and it transforms water. Kun (in the Eight Trigrams) corresponds to the west-south, earth, spleen primary Qi channel, and it

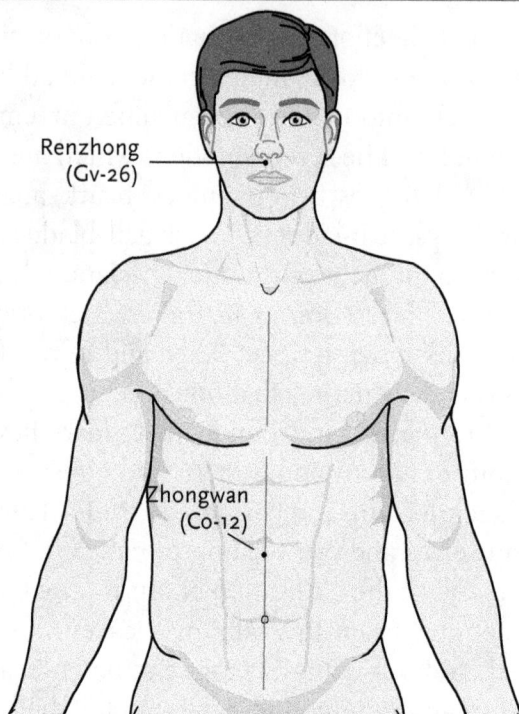

Figure 10. Renzhong (Gv-26) and
Zhongwan (Co-12) cavities

transforms earth. Xun (in the Eight Trigrams) corresponds to the east-south, gall bladder primary Qi channel, wood, and it transforms earth. Gen (in the Eight Trigrams) corresponds to the east-north, stomach primary Qi channel, earth, and it transforms fire. These are the internal Eight Trigrams. In terms of external Eight Trigrams, the number two and four are shoulders, six and eight are feet, above is nine and below is one, left is three and right is seven. Kan is one, Kun is two, Zhen is three, Xun is four, center is five, Qian is six, Dui is seven, Gen is eight, Li is nine, these are the nine palaces. The internal nine palaces are as such. In terms of external and internal (of a human body), Yi (in the Celestial Stem) corresponds to liver, left side of the ribs, transforms metal and communicates with the lungs. Jia (in the Celestial Stem) corresponds to gall bladder, transforms earth and communicates with the spleen.

Chengjiang
(Co-24)

Dihe
(M-HN-19)

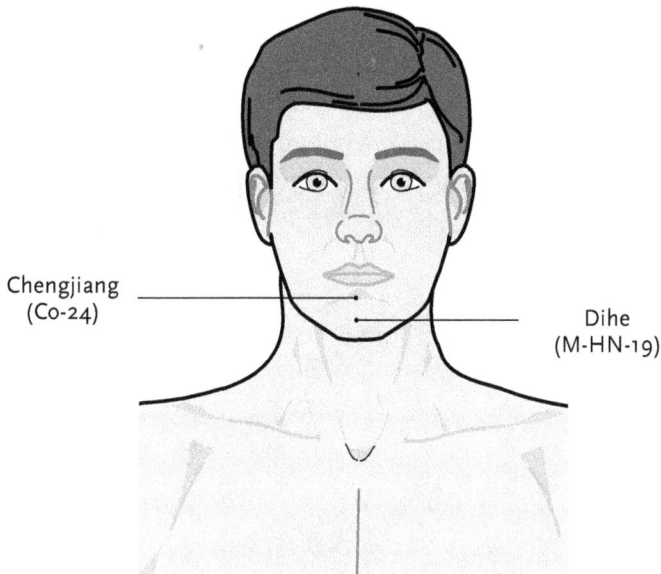

Figure 11. Dihe (M-HN-19) and
Chengjiang (Co-24) cavities

*Ding (in the Celestial Stem) corresponds to heart,
transforms wood and communicates with the liver. Bing
(in the Celestial Stem) corresponds to small intestine,
transforms water and communicates with the kidneys. Ji
(in the Celestial Stem) corresponds to spleen, transforms earth and communicates with the stomach. Shu
(in the Celestial Stem) corresponds to stomach, transforms fire and communicates with the heart. The rear
back and the front chest, Qi communicates in the
mountain and rivers. Xin (in the Celestial Stem) corresponds to lungs, side ribs on the right, transforms water
and communicates with kidneys, Geng (in the Celestial
Stem) corresponds to large intestine, transforms metal
and communicates with lungs, Gui (in the Celestial
Stem) corresponds to the lower part of the kidneys,
transforms fire and communicates with heart, Ren (in*

the Celestial Stem) corresponds to bladder, transforms water and communicates with liver. These are the internal and external correspondences of the Ten Celestial Stems. The Twelve Terrestrial Branches also have their internal and external correspondences. (If you) know these rules, then can (we) talk about the Dao of cultivating the body.

夫離南正午火心經，坎北正子水腎經，震東正卯木肝經，
兌西正酉金肺經，乾西北隅金大腸化水，坤西南隅土脾
化土，巽東南隅膽木化土，艮東北隅胃土化火，此內八
卦者，二四為肩，六八為足，上九下一，左三右七也。
坎一，坤二，震三，巽四，中五，乾六，兌七，艮八，
離九，此九宮也。內九宮亦如此。表裡者，乙肝左肋化
金通肺，甲膽化土通脾，丁心化木通肝，丙小腸化水通
腎，己脾化土通胃，戊胃化火通心，後背前胸，山澤通
氣，辛肺右肋化水通腎，庚大腸化金通肺，癸腎下部化
火通心，壬膀胱化水通肝，此十天干之內外也。十二地
支亦如此之內外也。明斯理，則可與言修身之道矣。

Nine palaces (Jiu Gong, 九宮) means nine assigned numbers for nine different locations (i.e., palaces) which correspond externally to the Eight Trigrams and also the center. Of the nine palaces, two and four (the second and fourth trigrams) are shoulders, six and eight are feet, above is nine and below is one, left is three and right is seven (Figure 12). When they correspond with the Eight Trigrams, Kan (坎)

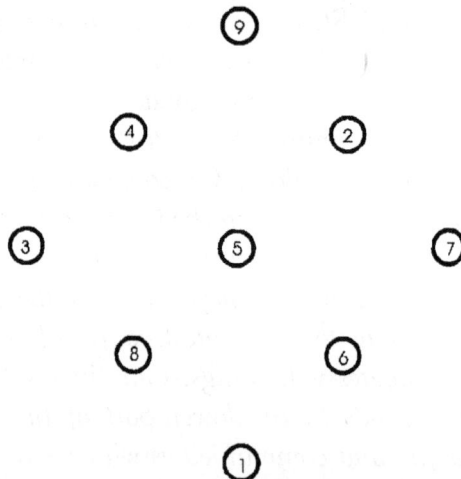

Figure 12. Locations of "Nine Palaces"

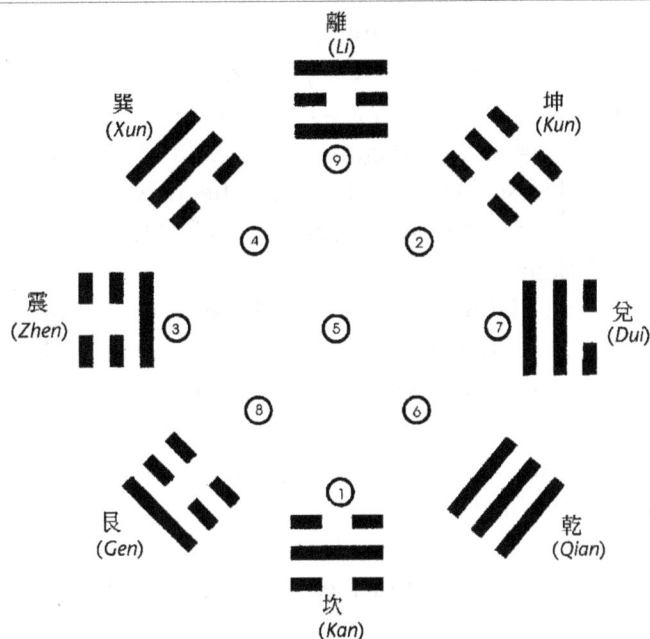

Figure 13. "Nine Palaces" and Eight Trigrams (Bagua)

is one, Kun (坤) is two, Zhen (震) is three, Xun (巽) is four, center (中) is five, Qian (乾) is six, Dui (兑) is seven, Gen (艮) is eight, Li (離) is nine, these are the nine palaces (Figure 13). The Eight Trigrams are related to the directions, time of the day, and different internal organs. For example, Li (離) in the Eight Trigrams corresponds to the south, Wu (午) in the Terrestrial (i.e., 11 A.M.-1 P.M.), fire, and heart primary Qi channel. Kan (坎) in the Eight Trigrams corresponds to the north, Zi (子) in the Terrestrial (i.e., 11 P.M.-1 A.M.), water, and kidney primary Qi channel. Zhen (震) in the Eight Trigrams corresponds to the east, Mao (卯) in the Terrestrial (i.e., 5-7 A.M.), fire, and heart primary Qi channel. Dui (兑) in the Eight Trigrams corresponds to the west, Qiu (酉) in the Terrestrial (i.e., 5-7 P.M.), metal, and lung primary Qi channel. Qian (乾) in the Eight Trigrams corresponds to the west-north, metal, large intestine primary Qi channel, and it transforms water. Kun (坤) in the Eight Trigrams corresponds to the west-south, earth, spleen primary Qi channel, and it transforms earth. Xun (巽) in the Eight Trigrams corresponds to the east-south, gall bladder primary Qi channel, wood, and it transforms earth. Gen (艮) in the Eight Trigrams corresponds to the east-north, stomach primary Qi channel, earth, and it transforms fire.

The Twelve Terrestrial Branches or Horary Characters (hourly characters) (Shi Er Di Zhi, 十二地支) are: Zi (子)(11 P.M.-1 A.M.)-Rat, Chou (丑)(1-3 A.M.)-Ox, Yin (寅)(3-5 A.M.)-Tiger, Mao (卯)(5-7 A.M.)-Hare, Chen (辰)(7-9 A.M.)-Dragon, Yi (巳)(9-11A.M.)-Snake, Wu (午)(11A.M.-1 P.M.)-Horse, Wei (未)(1-3 P.M.)-Sheep, Shen (申)(3-5 P.M.)-Monkey, Qiu (酋)(5-7 P.M.)-Cock, Shu (戌)(7-9 P.M.)-Dog, and Hai (亥)(9-11 P.M.)-Boar.

The term Celestial Stem implies a believed astrological influence, and is possibly a reference to the timing of techniques. In terms of external and internal correspondence of a human body, Yi (乙) in the Celestial Stem corresponds to liver, left side of the ribs, transforms metal and communicates with the lungs. Jia (甲) in the Celestial Stem corresponds to gall bladder, transforms earth and communicates with the spleen. Ding (丁) in the Celestial Stem corresponds to heart, transforms wood and communicates with the liver. Bing (丙) in the Celestial Stem corresponds to small intestine, transforms water and communicates with the kidneys. Ji (己) in the Celestial Stem corresponds to spleen, transforms earth and communicates with the stomach. Shu (戊) in the Celestial Stem corresponds to stomach, transforms fire and communicates with the heart. The rear back and the front chest, Qi communicates in the mountain and rivers. Xin (辛) in the Celestial Stem corresponds to lungs, side ribs on the right, transforms water and communicates with kidneys, Geng (庚) in the Celestial Stem corresponds to large intestine, transforms metal and communicates with lungs, Gui (癸) in the Celestial Stem corresponds to the lower part of the kidneys, transforms fire and communicates with heart, Ren (壬) in the Celestial Stem corresponds to bladder, transforms water and communicates with liver. These are the internal and external correspondences of the Ten Celestial Stems.

The Ten Celestial Stems are (Shi Tian Gan, 十天干): Jia (甲), Yi (乙), Bing (丙), Ding (丁), Wu (戊), Ji (己), Geng (庚), Xin (辛), Ren (壬), Gui (癸). In which, Jia and Yi correspond with wood of the Five Elements, Bing and Jin correspond with fire of the Five Elements, Wu and Ji correspond with the earth of the Five Elements, Geng and Xin correspond with metal of the Five Elements, and Ren and Gui correspond with the water of the Five Elements.

3.19 The Interpretation of Taiji Three Achievements of Scholarship and Martial Arts

When (we) talk about Dao (of studying Taijiquan), there can't be any achievement without having (a) self cultivation of the body (i.e., both internal and external). However, these cultivations can be divided into three levels. Levels means (the level of) achievements. Top level means great achievement, low level means little achievement, while the middle level means the achievements of sincerity (i.e., study sincerely). Cultivation methods can be divided into three paths. However, their (final) success (i.e., achievement) remains one. The scholarship (i.e., internal understanding) is for internal cultivation while the martial arts are for external cultivation. Physical education (i.e., education of understanding the physical body) is internal while martial matter is an external (manifestation). The method of cultivation which (allows you to) successfully accomplish the goal both internally and externally and has led (you) to reach a great (level of) achievement, is the top level. If martial (capability) in martial arts is gained due to (only) the study of physical education (i.e., internal understanding), or the (internal understanding) in physical education is gained due to (only) the martial (capability) of martial arts, then it is the middle level. However, those who only know physical education and do not know how to enter (i.e., get involved in) martial arts training, or those who specialize only in martial arts and do not know physical education, and have achieved the goal, are low level.

蓋言道者，非自修身無由得成也。然又分三乘之修法，乘者成也。上乘即大成也，下乘即小成也，中乘即誠之者成也。法分三修，成功一也。文修于內，武修于外，體育內也，武事外也。其修法，內外表裡成功，集大成即上乘也；由體育之文而得武事之武，或由武事之武而得體育之文，即中乘也；然獨知體育不入武事而成者，或專武事不為體育而成者，即下乘也。

The Dao of practicing Taijiquan can be divided into two aspects; the Yin internal aspect and the Yang external aspect. The Yin side includes the internal understanding of the Taiji theories, rules, and principles as well as understanding how the body works. The Yang side is to manifest and apply this internal comprehension and physical understanding into martial arts actions. How effectively Taiji martial arts are manifested externally depends on how much you understand the theories and the principles internally.

If you wish to achieve a high level and great achievement in Taijiquan art, you must study the theories, rules, and principles, ponder them deeply and comprehend the internal essence of the art profoundly. Moreover, you must also understand how to condition your body to allow you to manifest your Taiji martial techniques to their maximum efficiency and effectiveness.

If you practice Taijiquan with a deep and profound understanding of the theories and principles, and from this understanding gradually grasp the external martial capabilities, then you will have reached the middle level. If you practice only the physical movements and some shallow level of martial skills, and from this practice, you figure out some of the Taiji theory and principles, then you will only have reached the middle level.

However, if you practice Taijiquan only through study and understanding of the theories, rules, and principles, even if you do understand your body to a proper level, if you do not know how to manifest this internal understanding into martial actions, then you have only reached a low level. Similarly, if you practice Taijiquan only focusing on the martial aspects, without deeply pondering and understanding the theories, then the martial manifestation will also be shallow. In this case, you have reached only the lowest level.

3.20 The Interpretation of Taiji's Lower Level Martial Aspects

The martial aspects of Taijiquan are: the external oper- ations (i.e., actions) are gentle and soft while internally it contains the strength and hardness at the same time demanding the gentleness and softness internally. When gentleness and softness are manifested external- ly, after (practicing) for a long long time, then is able to be strong and hard internally. This is not caused due to the intention to be strong and hard, as a matter of fact, the intention is to be gentle and soft. What is the most difficult (thing to do) is to contain and store the strength and hardness internally without being applied (externally) while extremely gentle and soft when encountering the opponent. Use the gentleness and soft- ness to respond with the strength and hardness and make the (opponent's) strength and hardness dissolved into nothingness. But how can (we) achieve this goal? (You) must have accomplished the training of attach- ing, adhering, connecting, and following and be able to feel the movement sensitively, then (you) have gained Understanding Jin, afterwards, you can reach the enlightenment spiritually. (When this happens), (your) neutralization has reached an extremely high level. If (you) do not know the marvelousness of using four ounces to repel a thousand pounds and the achieve- ment is not yet reaching the level of neutralization, then how can (you) reach (the final goal of practice)? This is what is called, "understanding the attachment of the movements" until (you) have gained the tricky keys to sensitivity in seeing and listening (i.e., skin feeling).

太極下乘武事解

太極之武事，外操柔軟，內含堅剛而求柔軟。柔軟之于
外，久而久之，自得內之堅剛，非有心之堅剛，實有心
之柔軟也。所難者，內要含蓄堅剛而不施，外終柔軟而
迎敵，以柔軟而應堅剛，使堅剛盡化無有矣。其功何以
得乎？要非粘、黏、連、隨已成，自得運動知覺，方為
懂勁，而後神而明之，化境極矣。夫四兩撥千斤之妙，
功不及化境，將何以能是？所謂懂粘運得其視聽輕靈之
巧耳。

When Taiji martial arts are in action, the external movements are extremely soft. However, the internal mind and spirit which are used to lead the Qi must be strong. When the mind is strong, the Qi led will be abundant and the power manifested will naturally be powerful. Even though it is powerful, it is still soft. When you are soft, then are you able to apply the techniques of attaching, sticking, connecting, and following skillfully to neutralize the coming force. Naturally, executing these techniques effectively depends on the sensitivity of Listening Jin (i.e., skin feeling) with the assistance of the eyes' viewing and the ears' listening. Any Taijiquan beginner should aim for these training criteria. Once you have achieved this goal, then you have completed the lower level of Taijiquan practice.

3.21 The Interpretation of Taiji's Orthodox Practice

What is Taiji? It is round. It does not matter it is internal or external, up or down, left or right, it will not part from this roundness. What is Taiji? It is square. It does not matter it is internal or external, up or down, left or right, it will not (be) apart from this squareness. Enter and exit with the roundness, advance and retreat with the squareness. Follow the squareness and harmonize with the roundness for back and forth. Squareness is for opening and extensive (movements) while roundness is for tight and compact (actions). Roundness and squareness are the normative standards. What else could be apart from this standard? When this happens, (you) can move (your hands) as gaining the heart (i.e., move as wished), to reach the high and to drill the strong, be subtler and subtler, visible but seems invisible, brighter and brighter, continue forever without the end which cannot be stopped.

太極者，元（圓）也，無論內外上下左右，不離此元也；太極者，方也，無論內外上下左右，不離此方也。元之出入，方之進退，隨方就元之往來也。方為開展，元為緊湊，方元規矩之至，其孰能出此以外哉？如此得心應手，仰高鑽堅，神乎其神，見隱顯微，明而且明，生生不已，欲罷不能。

The Taiji in Taijiquan is the mind. This mind can generate roundness in action and strategies, and this mind can also produce square movements and maneuvers. Round is considered to be Yin in Taijiquan, which allows you to be soft and therefore can lead and neutralize the incoming force. Square is considered to be Yang, in which the actions are straight without hesitation, allowing you to move swiftly and with power. Soft is Yin while hard is Yang. Knowing Yin and Yang, then can you say you know Taijiquan.

When you are round, not only can you lead and neutralize the incoming strong force, but you can also, through coiling action, approach your opponent's center. When you are square, due to the straight and speedy action, you can advance, retreat, and move to the side with appropriate speed and timing. The square actions are wide open and extended, while the round maneuvers are more compact and executed in a closer range. Only if you can use these two Yin and Yang concepts skillfully, can you then easily exchange insubstantial and substantial as you wish. From this achievement, you can then reach a proficient level of Taijiquan applications.

3.22 The Interpretation of Taiji's Lightness, Heaviness, Floating, and Sinking

The fault of double weighting is related to overdoing and is different from (double) sinking. Double sinking is not a fault since it is agile and nimble, and it is not the same as heaviness. Double floating is a fault since it is drifting and distant, and it is not the same as lightness. Double lightness is not a fault since it is light and agile naturally, and it is not the same as floating. Half lightness and half heaviness is not a fault, however too much of lightness or heaviness is a fault. When there is a half, means there is a final goal (i.e., reason or purpose) to be half, therefore, it is not a fault. When there is too much emphasis (either in lightness or heaviness), because there is no final goal (i.e., reason or purpose) to have too much emphasis, therefore, it is a fault. When there is too much emphasis without a reason, then it must have parted from the square and round (actions). When there is a half and there is a reason for it, how can it be parted from square and round (actions)? (However,) half floating or half sinking is a fault, it is an error due to insufficient (effort). When there is too much of floating or too much of sinking, then it is a fault due to too excessive. If there is a half heaviness or too much of heaviness, then it is stagnant and not upright. If there is half lightness or too much of lightness, then though it is agile, it loses roundness. When there is half sinking or too much of sinking, then insubstantial and not upright. If there is half floating or too much of floating, then confused without roundness.

太極輕、重、浮、沉解

雙重為病，干于填施，與沉不同也；雙沉不為病，自爾
騰虛，與重不易也。雙浮為病，只如漂渺，與輕不例也；
雙輕不為病，天然清靈，與浮不等也。半輕半重不為病；
偏輕偏重為病。半者，半有著落也，所以不為病；偏者，
偏無著落也，所以為病。偏無著落，必失方圓；半有著
落，豈出方圓？半浮半沉為病，失于不及也；偏浮偏沉，
失于太過也。半重偏重，滯而不正也；半輕偏輕，靈而
不圓也。半沉偏沉，虛而不正也；半浮偏浮，茫而不圓
也。

Double weighting means when the opponent has placed a force (i.e., weight) on you, you react with a force or weight. This is an action of mutual resistance. When this happens, the Qi and actions will become stagnant, and the maneuvers of lightness and agility will become hard to execute easily. Once you have lost your lightness and agility, you will not be able to apply the strategies of insubstantial and substantial.

However, how does double weighting happen? First, you must understand that double sinking is different from double weighting. Double sinking is a strategy and has a legitimate purpose, while double weighting serves no purpose but is simply a product of mindless resistance. You must understand that the sinking here means the sinking of the force, instead of a physical sinking of the body. This sinking force comes from Growing Jin (Zhang Jin, 長勁). When you apply double sinking to your opponent, you are soft and already have a firm root, which allows you to destroy the opponent's center, balance, and root. However, when you are in a double weighting situation, you will be floating and stiff, which allows your opponent to find your root. You might already have a firm root, and even be soft, but if you react with too much blind force, it will produce double weighting. But if you apply your force appropriately, then it will produce sinking. When you are in a double weighting situation, you are stiff, struggling, and stagnant. However, if you are in a double sinking situation, you can be agile and nimble.

By similar analysis, floating is not the same as lightness. If in response to incoming force, your force is too light, it is floating. When this happens, your force is insufficient, drifting and distant, which makes it difficult for you to sense the opponent's action and further reach the opponent's center. However, if your contact is light and appropriate, you can be agile, which allows you to sense the opponent's intention (i.e., Listening Jin) and neutralize it.

If the force you apply is neither too light nor too heavy (i.e., appropriate), then it is not a fault. This is simply because each technique is also a set up for further action. This can also be expressed by the feeling of one side of your body's action being light while the other side is heavy. When this happens, you can exchange insubstantial and substantial maneuvers easily. However, if one side is too light and/or the other side is too heavy, then it is a fault because the inappropriate application of force can be used by your opponent. If the force and strategies are correct, you can be square or round without stagnation as you wish.

However, half floating and half sinking, and also half heaviness or even too much sinking are all faults. This is because they can cause deficiency or excess of the action. It is the same whether there is half lightness or too much lightness, half sinking or too much sinking, half floating or too much floating—all will deprive you of your agility, roundness, center, and root.

If double lightness but not becoming floating, then there is lightness and agility; (if) double sinking but not becoming heaviness, then is apart from deceptiveness (i.e., is firmed). Therefore, it is said: "The top hands (i.e., highest skills)(know) lightness and heaviness. Those (who know) half (heaviness or lightness) are average hand (i.e., skill)." Other than these three, all are faults. This is because when the insubstantial and agility are not vague (i.e., clear) internally, it can result in the clarity and brightness of the external Qi circulating in the four limbs. If (you) do not thoroughly study the techniques of lightness, heaviness, floating, and sinking, then (you will) sigh as if (you are) digging a well without being able to reach the spring. However, if (you have) the skills of squareness, roundness, and the four sides, which can be manifested externally, internally, fine, and coarse as wished, then (you) have approached the great achievement. How can it still be said that the four corners are departed from the squareness and roundness? This is what is said "from the squareness to the roundness and from the roundness to the square-ness, which are beyond the appearance. In this case, (you) have reached the highest hands (i.e., skills) of the ultimate transcendence."

夫雙輕不近于浮，則有輕靈；雙沉不近于重，則為離虛。
故曰：上手輕重，半有著落，則為平手。除此三者之外，
皆為病手。蓋內虛靈不昧，能致于外氣之清明，流行乎
肢體也。若不窮研輕重浮沉之手，徒勞掘井不及泉之嘆
耳。然有方圓四正之手，表里精粗無不到，則已極大成，
又何云四隅出方圓矣？所謂方而圓，圓而方，超乎象外，
得其寰中之上手也。

If you can achieve double lightness without it becoming floating, then you can be light and agile. If you can achieve double sinking without it becoming heaviness, then you will have a firm root. From the discussion above, we can see that "double lightness," "double heaviness," and "half heaviness and half lightness" are not faults. Those people who know how to apply double heaviness and lightness are the proficient ones. However, those who know only half heaviness and half lightness are the average skill practitioners. Mindful, deep and consistent practice is required over a long time.

This is because if your mind is clear in what you are doing, then you can be agile and your actions can be alive. When this happens, the Qi can be led by the mind smoothly, and can be externally manifested efficiently. Therefore, in order to reach a profound level of Taijiquan practice, a practitioner must always study and ponder the theory of lightness and heaviness. Only when this understanding has been manifested externally can you be round and also be square. In this case, you have grasped the crucial keys to Taijiquan combat.

3.23 The Interpretation of Taiji's Four Corners

Four cardinal directions are four sides, and are what are called Peng, Lu, Ji, and An. If at beginning, (you) do not know (the concept of) how the squareness can be applied to roundness and the theory of the ceaseless repeating cycle of the squareness and roundness, then how (can you) derive the skills of the four corners? This is related to our external limbs and internal spirit and Qi. If (you are) not able to seize (i.e., accomplish) the skills of lightness, agility, squareness, and roundness, also avoid the faults of lightness, heaviness, floating, and sinking how can (you) derive four corners. For example, (if you commit a) half heaviness or too much of heaviness, then (your skills) are stagnant and (body) disordered. Naturally, you will use the skills of four corners—Cai, Lie, Zhou, and Kao. Alternatively, (if you commit) a double weightedness and becoming an excessive fullness, (then) you will also apply the four corners techniques. (When you) have too many faulty skills, without choice, (you) must rely on the skills of four corners to compensate it, then (are you) able to return to the skills of proper roundness and squareness. Even though, those practitioners with low skills must rely on the Zhou and Kao to compensate (their deficiencies). After practicing for a long time, those whose Gongfu has reached to the top skills, must also acquire (the skills of) Cai and Lie to reach a high level of correctness and righteousness. That means the applications of the four corners are to be used to compensate (for) the deficiency of the main part of the art (i.e., four sides).

太
極
四
隅
解

四正即四方也，所謂掤、攦、擠、按也。初不知方能使圓，方圓復始之理無已，焉能出隅之手矣。緣人外之肢體，內之神氣，弗緝輕靈方圓四正之功，始出輕重浮沉之病，則有隅矣。譬如半重偏重，滯而不正，自然為采、挒、肘、靠之隅手，或雙重填實，亦出隅手也。病多之手，不得已以隅手扶之，而歸圓中方正之手。雖然，至低者肘靠，亦及此以補其所以云爾。舂後功夫能致上乘者，亦須獲采、挒而仍歸大中至正矣。是四隅之所用者，因失體而補缺云云。

Peng (掤)(i.e., Wardoff), Lu (攦)(i.e., Rollback), Ji (擠)(i.e., Press), and An (按)(i.e., Push) are the four main Jin patterns of Taijiquan which build up the most important foundation of Taijiquan. Most beginners do not know how to apply and exchange the strategies of roundness and squareness skillfully, and consequently they are not able to apply the Jin patterns of four corners, which include: Cai (采)(i.e., Pluck), Lie (挒)(i.e., Split), Zhou (肘)(i.e., Elbow), and Kao (靠)(i.e., Bump). In order to apply the roundness and squareness and avoid the faults of too light, heavy, floating, and sinking, you must first learn how to harmonize and coordinate your internal and external. Only then can you use your spirit and mind to lead the Qi for external manifestation. However, it is not easy to reach this goal for a beginner. In order to compensate for these faults, the Jin patterns of four corners are adopted. Because of the help of the four corners, you can apply roundness and squareness in your techniques.

However, you should not misunderstand that the four corners Jin patterns are only used for beginners. In fact, even after you have reached to a proficient level in the Jin patterns of the four cardinal directions, the four corners Jin patterns are still critical in your applications. Without the four corners, your Taijiquan techniques and skills will not be complete.

3.24 The Interpretation of Taiji's Balance, Waist, and the Head's Upward Suspension

The crown (of the head) is just like the plumb line (of a balance), therefore, it is said: "the head is suspended from above." Both hands are the trays on the left and right of the balance. The waist is like the root and stem of the balance. If (your) standing posture is like a balance, then even slightly off of what are called "lightness, heaviness, floating, or sinking," will be obvious. There is a plumb line from Weilu (i.e., tailbone) to the Xinmen (i.e., crown) which makes the head suspended and the waist as stem firmly connected to the root.

頂如準，故云頂頭懸也。兩手即平左右之盤也，腰即平之根株也。立如平準，所謂輕重浮沉，分厘毫絲則偏顯然矣。有準頂頭懸，腰之根下株，尾閭至囟門也。

When you practice Taijiquan, your torso should be upright. That means the crown is suspended upward. The torso, especially the waist, should be soft and centered, and the tailbone is tucked under. When this happens, your entire body will be connected, centered, and rooted. This center is just like the plumb line of a balance. Once you have firmed this central line, both of your hands, like the trays at the ends of a scale, can react naturally and gracefully. Xinmen (囟門) is located at the crown of the head. Next is a passage about this central line.

From the top to the bottom are connected as a line, (the actions) are all relying on the turning of the two arms on the balance. Variations and exchange (of the techniques) are measured according to centimeter and millimeter (i.e., refined) and you must discriminate the foot and inch (i.e., carefully) by yourself. Two Mingmen (i.e., kidneys) are like car wheels. When the flag waves (i.e., signaled), they shake and turn. When the Xin (i.e.,

太極平、準、腰、頂解

mind) gives an order, the Qi immediately follows. Then (you) can execute (your) actions as you wish naturally. The entire body must be light and agile. Train the body to become a steel Arhan. There are back and forth in sparring, sooner or later (will you become familiar with these skills). When there is a closing (i.e., storing the Jin), (the Jin) immediately emits. (When you execute Jin efficiently), the emitting arrow (i.e., Jin) does not have to reach to the sky (i.e., far). How much of the composure (you have) allows (you) to repel (the opponent) far with a single breathing with the sound of Ha. (The above secrets) must be secretly transmitted orally. This allows (you) to open the gate to see the heaven (i.e., comprehend suddenly or become enlightened).

上下一條線，全憑兩平轉。變換取分毫，尺寸自己辨。
車輪兩命門，一蠡搖又轉。心令氣旗使，自然隨我便。
滿身輕利者，金剛羅漢煉。對待有往來，是早或是晚。
合則放發去，不必凌霄箭。涵養有多少，一氣哈而遠。
口授秘傳，開門見中天。

When you have an upright and balanced center, you can turn your body as you wish without tilting. In this case, you can control the situation and control even the slightest change. Mingmen (命門) here means the two kidneys. This implies the waist area. Therefore, the waist is the place which directs the action. It is said in the *Taiji Classic* that: "The root is at the feet, (Jin or movement is) generated from the legs, mastered (i.e., controlled) by the waist and manifested (i.e., expressed) from the fingers." From this classic, we can see that when you keep your center and balance, you can control your waist easily with your mind (Xin, 心). When you are tilted, your mind will be scattered and confused. If you do not have a calm and clear mind to make good judgments, the Qi cannot be led to the desired place for effective manifestation.

In addition, when you are balanced and centered, your body can be loose and soft. This allows you to act with lightness and agility. This can also provide you with a great opportunity to be hard (square) or soft (round) as you wish. How capable you are of defeating your opponent depends on how much Gongfu (功夫) you have put into your skills. The two sounds of Hen (哼) and Ha (哈) can help you store and emit your Jin to its maximum level. The secret of using the Hen and Ha sound for manifesting Jin must be learned in person from a qualified master. Once you have grasped this secret, you will be enlightened immediately on this subject.

太極四時五氣解圖

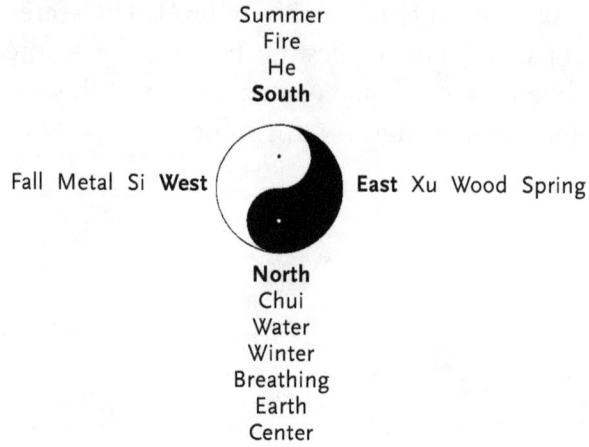

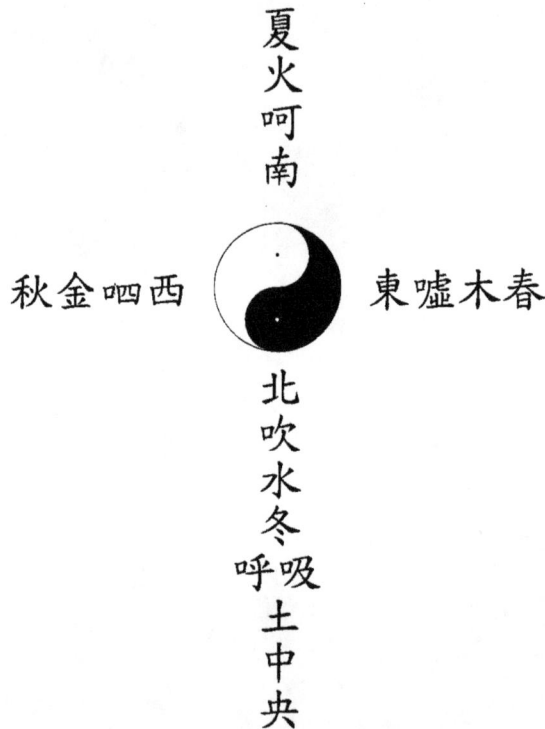

3.25 The Illustration of Taiji's Four Seasons and Five Qis

```
                    Summer
                    Fire
                    He
                    South

Fall  Metal  Si  West   ☯   East  Xu  Wood  Spring

                    North
                    Chui
                    Water
                    Winter
                    Breathing
                    Earth
                    Center
```

夏
火
呵
南

秋金呬西　☯　東噓木春

北
吹
水　　吸
冬
呼
土
中
央

3.26 Interpretation of the Foundation in Taiji's Blood and Qi

The blood is (used for) managing (the life) while Qi is to guard (the health of the body). The blood circulates (strongly) in the flesh, fasciae, and arms while the Qi circulates (abundantly) in the bones, tendons, and vessels. The tendons and nails are the superfluity of the bones, and the hairs are the superfluity of the blood. When the blood's circulation is abundant, then the hairs flourish. When the Qi is sufficient, then the tendons and nails are strong. The applicable functions of the Qi and blood are manifested in the inner strength of the flesh, fasciae, and nails. (The condition of) Qi relies on the sufficiency or insufficiency of the blood, and (the condition of) the blood depends on the Qi's rising or falling. This rising and falling, sufficiency and insufficiency are repeated from the beginning after completion of a cycle. This provides (us) the supply (of the Qi and blood) for entire life without exhaustion.

血為營，氣為衛，血流行于肉、膜、胳，氣流行于骨、筋、脈。筋甲為骨之餘，髮毛為血之餘，血旺則髮毛盛，氣足則筋甲壯。氣血之體用，出于肉、筋、甲之內壯。氣以血之盈虛，血以氣之消長，消長盈虛，周而復始，終身用之，不能盡者矣。

According to Chinese medicine, blood is the material that carries the Qi, nutrition, and other required material for the physical body's growth and functioning. When the blood's circulation is abundant and smooth, the muscles, fasciae, and four limbs will be healthy and strong. When the Qi's circulation is abundant and strong in the eight vessels, the bones and tendons will be strong. Qi exists around the entire body and even beyond the physical body, forming an energy shield to guard the body (Guardian Qi)(i.e., Wei Qi, 衛氣). It is believed that from the hair and the fingernails' growing condition, we can make a judgment whether the blood and the Qi are circulating abundantly and smoothly in the body. This is because the condition of the blood and Qi circulation in the body is manifested externally and shown in the appearance of the hairs and fingernails (e.g., color, smoothness, luster, clarity). Blood and Qi mutually support each other. When one is abundant, the other follows and when one is deficient, the other will also be affected. This kind of persistent, mutual influence in the body we perceive as a cycle. This circulation cycle is often affected by the time of the day (i.e., by the sun), the month (i.e., by the moon), by the seasons, and other long term natural heavenly cycles. For example, according to Chinese medicine, the main Qi circulation in the twelve internal organs is affected by the time of day. This is called "midnight, noon, major Qi flow" (Zi Wu Liu Zhu, 子午流注). Similarly, our bodily Qi circulation is also influenced by other natural powers or forces which fall upon us.

3.27 The Interpretation of Taiji's Li and Qi

太
極
力
氣
解

The Qi is circulating in the fasciae, arms (i.e., limbs), tendons, and vessels, and the Li (i.e., muscular force) is originated from blood, flesh, skin, and bones. Therefore, those who have Li manifest their strength in the skin and bones. This belongs to the shape (i.e., physical form). Those who have (abundant) Qi manifest the inner strength in the tendons and vessels. This belongs to the appearance (i.e., feeling of phenomenon). The Qi-blood is applied to the inner strength while blood-Qi is used for external strength. (If you) understand the function of the Qi and blood, then (you) can understand the origin of the Li and Qi (i.e., Jin). (If you) know the natural (functions) of the Qi and Li, then (you) can distinguish the difference of using the Li and circulating the Qi. To circulate the Qi in the tendons and fasciae and to apply the Li in the skin and bones are very different.

氣走于膜、胳、筋、脈，力出于血、肉、皮、骨。故有力者皆外壯于皮骨，形也；有氣者是內壯于筋脈，象也。氣血功用于內壯，血氣功用于外壯。要之明于〝氣血〞二字之功能，自知力氣之由來矣。知氣力之所以然，自能用力行氣之分別，行氣于筋脈，用力于皮骨，大不相侔也。

According to the contemporary model of Qi as bioelectricity, the fasciae and skin are poor electrical conductors, while the tendons and muscles are good conductors that can transport the Qi strongly and smoothly. The tendons have higher electrical conductivity than the muscles; therefore, the muscles will trap the Qi and manifest it into physical force (i.e., Li, 力). However, when the muscles are relaxed and the tendons are used to manifest the Qi into physical forms, they are soft while the Qi is strong. When this happens, the Taiji Jin (i.e., soft Jin) can be manifested as a soft whip. This soft Jin can be penetrating, while the muscular Li, though powerful, will generate power that is only shallow. When Qi is focused and manifested into physical forms, it is Jin. However, if your power is manifested only through the blood circulation that carries the Qi to the muscles, then it is Li. Therefore, in Taijiquan practice, you must focus on the Qi's development and circulation. That is why Taijiquan is an internal martial art and Qigong practice.

3.28 The Interpretation of Taiji's Meter, Decimeter, Centimeter, and Millimeter

(Practicing Taiji) Gongfu should first train opening and expanding and then train tightness and compactness. When the (practice of) opening and expanding have achieved their results (i.e., goals), then should (we) talk about tightness and compactness. When the tightness and compactness have been accomplished, then should (we) talk about the foot, inch, centimeter, and millimeter (Jins). After (you) have achieved the result of the foot (Jin), then should (you) be able to pursue the inch, centimeter, and millimeter (Jins). This (concept) is clear when (we) talk about the principle of the meter, decimeter, centimeter, and millimeter. However, every meter must have ten decimeters, every decimeter must have ten centimeters, and every centimeter must have ten millimeters. Its number has been defined. Therefore, when (you) match (i.e., spar) with (your opponent), (we) talk about numbers. When (you) know the number, then (you) can master the skills of foot, inch, centimeter, and millimeter (Jins). In order to know these numbers, how can (you) reach this capability without a secret teaching?

功夫先練開展，後練緊湊。開展成而得之，才講緊湊。
緊湊得成，才講尺寸分毫。由尺住之功成，而後能寸住、
分住、毫住，此所謂尺寸分毫之理也明矣。然尺必十寸，
寸必十分，分必十毫，其數在焉。故云對待者數也。知
其數，則能得尺寸分毫也。要知其數，非秘授而能量之
者哉！

Gongfu (功夫) means "energy-time" in Chinese. That implies that any study or practice which takes a long time and great effort to accomplish is "Gongfu." To reach a proficient level of Taijiquan takes a great deal of effort and time, therefore, practicing Taijiquan is called "Gongfu."

太極尺、寸、分、毫解

When you practice Taijiquan, initially the postures and movements should be expansive and large. This allows you to be relaxed, comfortable, and soft so that the Qi can circulate smoothly. Only after you have reached a high level of relaxation and softness, can you then still be relaxed and soft even when the postures and movements are more compact and tighter.

The reason for this distance change is simply that, when you are in a more compact and tight posture, you are closer to your opponent. In this case, in order to neutralize any incoming force in such a short distance, your listening, attaching, adhering, connecting, and following Jins must have reached a profound level. In addition, it is easier to manifest your Jin from a longer distance than a shorter one. If the Jin manifested is not powerful, the attempt will be in vain. Naturally, you will be defeated by your opponent.

In order to achieve more compact, tight, close range Jin manifestation, you must first have a higher sensitivity in feeling (i.e., Listening Jin). Only then can you direct the Qi to the correct place for manifestation. Therefore, in order to reach a more compact fighting range for shorter Jin manifestation, you must start with the listening Jin training. When this feeling has improved and becomes more sensitive, then you can shorten your fighting range and Jin manifestation.

Generally in Taijiquan combat, a deep level Taijiquan fighter will try to keep the distance between himself and his opponent shorter. This will make it more difficult for the opponent to apply his techniques effectively and powerfully, while the Taiji fighter can still be effective in his execution of techniques.

3.29 The Interpretation of Fasciae, Vessels, Tendons, and Cavities

Controlling the fasciae, seizing the (Qi) vessels, grabbing the tendons, and sealing the cavities, these four Gong (i.e., Gongfu) are obtained (first) from (mastering the skills of) the foot, inch, centimeter, and millimeter Jins. Only then can they be pursued. (When) the fasciae are controlled, the blood will not be circulating completely; (when) the (Qi) vessels are seized, the Qi is hard to transport; (when) the tendons are grabbed, the body will lose its master (i.e., control); (when) the cavities are sealed, the spirit will be dizzy and the Qi is dark (i.e., fainting can occur). (When) fasciae are grabbed and controlled, (your opponent) will be as half dead; (when Qi) vessels are exposed and seized, (your opponent) will be as dead; (if) tendons can be grabbed singly, the (opponent's) Jin can be broken; (if) the death cavities are sealed, then there is no life. In all, if (the opponent) does not have Qi and blood('s circulation) and spirit of vitality, how can he still be the master of himself/herself? However, if (you wish) to achieve the Gong of controlling, seizing, grabbing, and sealing, (you) must have (a qualified master's) personal instruction.

節膜、拿脈、抓筋、閉穴，此四功由尺寸分毫得之，後而求之。膜若節之，血不周流；脈若拿之，氣難行走；筋若抓之，身無主地；穴若閉之，神昏氣暗。抓膜節之半死，申脈拿之似亡，單筋抓之勁斷，死穴閉之無生。總之氣血精神，若無身何有主也？如能節、拿、抓、閉之功，非得點傳不可。

There are four ultimate level fighting skills in Chinese martial arts training. These four skills are: controlling the fasciae (Jie Mo, 節膜), seizing the (Qi) vessels (Na Mai, 拿脈), grabbing the tendons (Zhua Jin, 抓筋), and sealing the cavities (Bi Xue, 閉穴). In order to execute these four skills effectively, you must first build up your sensitivity until it has reached a high level. Only then can you shorten

太極膜、脈、筋、穴解

your Jin from a foot to only a millimeter. Without the sensitive feeling and the accuracy of the execution of skills, you will not be able to reach this level. When the fasciae are controlled, it can affect the blood circulation. When the Qi vessels are seized, Qi circulation will become stagnant. When the tendons are grabbed, the opponent cannot move easily. When the cavities are sealed, the opponent can be made to faint or even be killed. Although these four skills are very effective in a fight, however, very few martial artists can reach this level. The reason for this is simply because the training of these four skills is normally kept secret by masters. Only very trusted students will be taught personally.

3.30 The Word by Word Interpretation of Taiji

太
極
字
字
解

> *To file, circle rub, pound, and strike (are related) [to myself or to the opponent]; to press down, scour, push, and control (are related)[to myself or to the opponent]; to open, close, rise, and fall (are related)[to myself or to the opponent], these twelve words are all using the hands. To bend, extend, move, and calm (are related) [to ourselves and to the opponent]; to ascend, descend, speed up, and slow down (are related) [to myself and to the opponent]; to dodge, return, scoop, and cease (are related) [to myself and to the opponent], these twelve words are talking about the Qi in ourselves and applying to the opponent. (Brackets in original.)*

挫、柔、捶、打〔于己、于人〕，按、摩、推、拿〔于
己、于人〕，開、合、升、降〔于己、于人〕，此十二
字皆用手也。屈、伸、動，靜〔于己、于人〕，起、落、
急、緩〔于己、于人〕，閃、還、撩、了〔于己、于
人〕，此十二字于己氣也，于人手也。

Filing (Cuo, 挫、搓) is a straight line action, using the forearm or the edge of the hand to file the opponent's body—for example, the side of the waist or the sides of the neck (Figure 14). It can also be used to break the joints, such as the elbow (Figure 15). Filing is a vital skill that is used to damage the opponent's fasciae (Jie Mo, 節膜). Circle rubbing (Rou, 柔、揉) is a circular rubbing action using the palm or the base of the palm to press the opponent and then rub in with circles. Circle rubbing is commonly used to damage the opponent's fasciae. It can also be used to attack the cavities with the knuckle of a finger—for example, the joint of the index finger is used to rub into the cavities (Figure 16). Pounding (Cui, 捶) is a strike from the top moving down that acts like a hammer's pounding. Striking (Da, 打) is a general straight forward punch.

Pressing downward (An, 按) is an action that uses the palm to press downward, used either to seal the arm's further action (Figure 17) or used against a vital area such as in a strike (Figure 18). Scouring (Mo, 摩) is a quick frictional movement on the opponent's

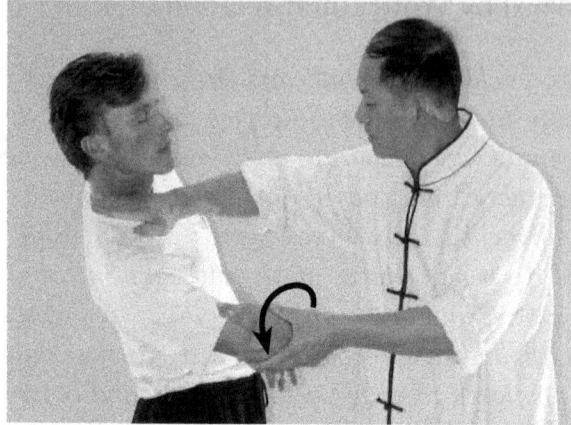

Figure 14. Using Cuo (i.e., filing) technique to attack the side of the neck

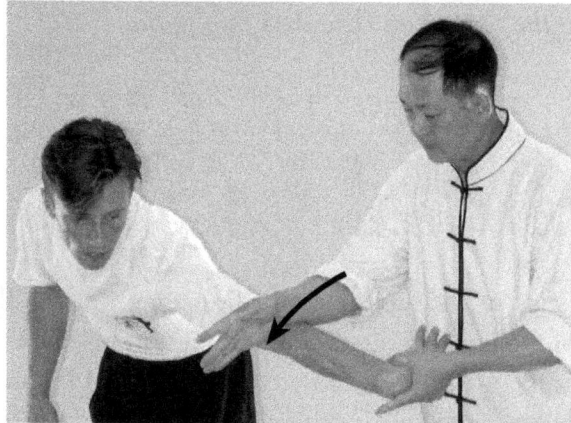

Figure 15. Using Cuo (i.e., filing) technique to break the elbow joint

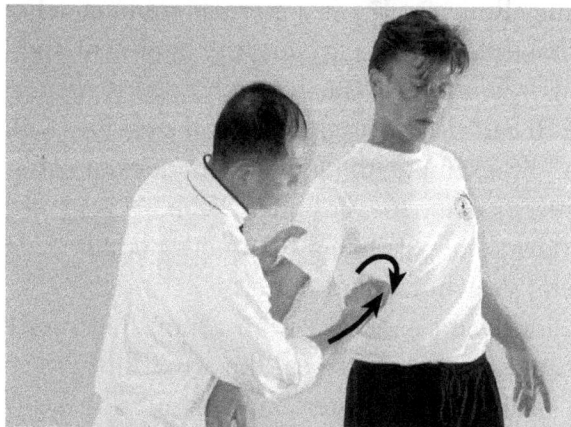

Figure 16. Using Rou (i.e., circle rubbing) technique to attack Qimen (Li-14) cavity

skin. This action allows you to move from one place to another without losing contact with the opponent. Pushing (Tui, 推) is an action using the palm to push forward, upward, or downward to the opponent's body. Controlling (Na, 拿) is using your hands to stick with the opponent's joints and control them (Figure 19). Na in Taijiquan is not an action of grabbing like in external styles. This is because when a grabbing action is initiated, you will be tensed. Therefore, Taijiquan prefers the skill of plucking (Cai, 採) instead of grabbing. In addition to the above eight words, the arms' or hands' opening (Kai, 開), closing (He, 合), raising (Sheng, 升), and falling (Jiang, 降), are all actions of the hands. These actions are initiated from you and are applied to the opponent.

Bending (Qu, 屈), extending (Shen, 伸), moving (Dong, 動), calming down (i.e., stillness)(Jing, 靜), ascending (Qi, 起), descending (Luo, 落), speeding up (Ji, 急), slowing down (Huan, 緩), dodging (Shan, 閃), returning (i.e., turning back)(Huan, 還), provoking (i.e., inciting)(Liao, 撩), and ceasing (Liao, 了 are the twelve Taijiquan key words that relate to the mind and the Qi. These are initiated from relative thinking (i.e., strategies) on yourself and your opponent. Liao (撩) means to cheat the opponent to induce his action.

To turn, exchange, advance, and retreat (apply)[to myself in relation to the opponent's steppings]; to look (to the left), beware of (the right), front, and rear (talk about)[my eyes in relation to the opponent's hands]. This is gazing to the front and peek to the rear, look to the left and beware of the right; these eight words are related to the spirit. To break, connect, lean forward, and bend backward, these four words are related to the Yi and Jin. Connecting is related to the spirit and the Qi, lead forward and bend backward are related to the hands and legs. The Jin can be broken and Yi cannot be broken. When the Yi is broken, the spirit can still make connection (effective). However, if Jin, Yi, and spirit are all broken, then bending forward or leaning backward,

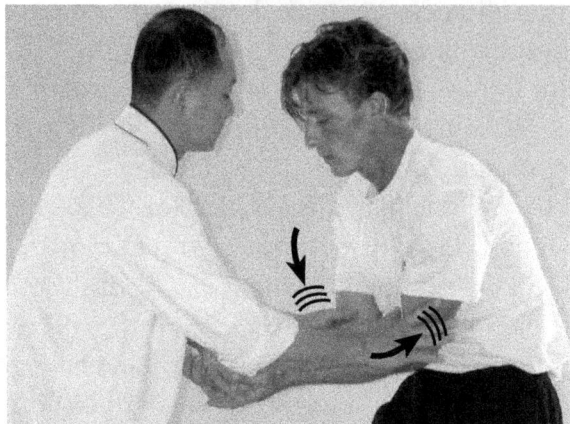

Figure 17. Using An (i.e., pressing down) to
seal the opponent's arm

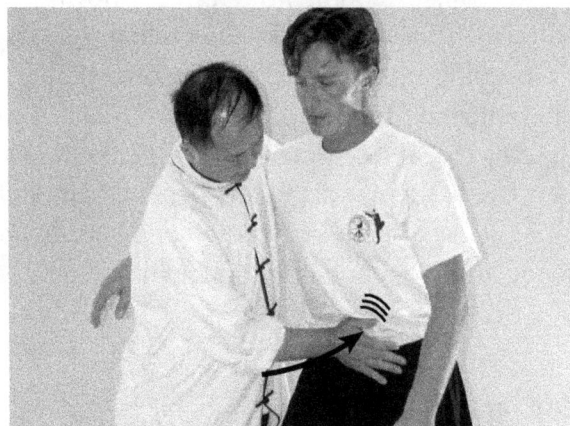

Figure 18. Using An (i.e., pressing) to strike the
Jiuwei cavity (Co-15)

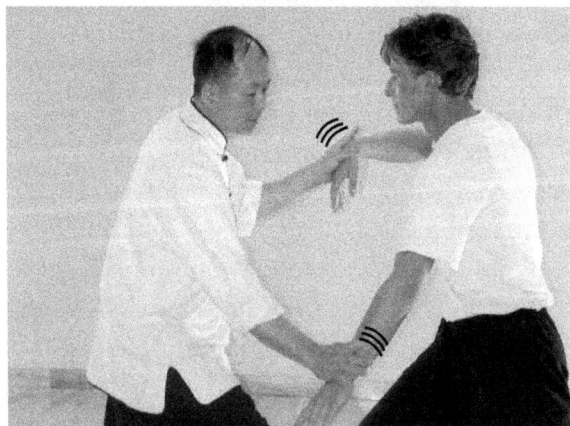

Figure 19. Using Na (i.e., controlling) to control
the opponent's wrist joints

and the hands and feet will have lost their positions.
Bending forward is bowing and bending backward
means reversing (i.e., reversed from bowing). To avoid
leaning forward and bending backward, the Jin must be
broken and reconnect. (Brackets in original.)

轉、換、進、退〔于己身、于人步也〕，顧、盼、前、
後〔于己目也、于人手也〕，即瞻前眇後，左顧右盼也，
此八字關乎神矣。斷、接、俯、仰，此四字關乎意勁也。
接關乎神氣也，俯仰關乎手足也，勁斷意不斷，意斷神
可接，勁意神俱斷，則俯仰矣，手足無著落耳。俯為一
叩，仰為一反而已矣。不使叩反，非斷而復接不可。

Turning (Zhuan, 轉), exchanging (Huan, 換), advancing forward (Jin, 進), and retreating backward (Tui, 退) are the four key
moving skills which allow you to correspond with the opponent's
stepping actions. Here, turning means to turn your body, while
exchanging implies exchanging your legs' positions. Pay attention to
the left (Zuo Gu, 左顧), beware of the right (You Pan, 右盼), gazing
to the front (Zhan Qian, 瞻前) and peeking to the rear (Miao Hou,
眇後), are the four key actions which bring you awareness and a high
level of alertness. Without these four awarenesses, your four body
moving skills will not be effective. All of these successes depend on
the alertness of your spirit.

Breaking (Duan, 斷), connecting (Jie, 接), leaning forward (Fu,
俯), and bending backward (Yang, 仰), are the four key words that
relate to the Yi (意)(i.e., mind) and Jin (勁). Whenever you change
your actions from offensive into defensive or vice versa, your Jin is
broken. When this happens, as long as your Yi is continuous, the broken Jin can be reconnected. You should remember that Yi is always
ahead of Jin. It is the Yi which leads the Qi to the physical body for
an action. Therefore, as long as Yi is not broken, the Jin can be reconnected. However, if the Yi is broken, then your mind will be scattered
and confused. When this happens, the broken Jin will be hard to
reconnect. Even in the worst situation, if you can keep your spirit in
a highly alert state, the Jin can be reconnected and the Yi can regain
calmness and continuity. However, if your Jin, Yi, and spirit are all

broken, then you will be bending forward and leaning backward. Therefore, you have lost your balance and centering. Your root will also be destroyed. When this happens, you will be surely defeated. To avoid bending forward and leaning backward, you must know how to reconnect whenever your Jin or Yi is broken.

In terms of sparring, (the problems of) bending forward and leaning backward must be taken seriously. Pay attention to the mind, body, hands, and feet and avoid being broken. (If you) do not know how to reconnect, then (you) are unable to bend forward and backward. In order to acquire the capability of broken and reconnecting, (you) must be able to see (i.e., comprehend) the hidden and subtle (action or Jin). When it is hidden and subtle, it is as broken as not broken. When it can be seen apparently, it seems connected but not connected. Connect and broken, broken and connect, (if you) can) conceal and manifest the Yi (i.e., wisdom mind), Xin (i.e., emotional mind), body, spirit, and Qi to their extreme level, how (can you) be afraid of not being able to attach, adhere, connect, and follow.

對待之字，以俯仰為重，時刻在心身手足，不使斷之。
無接則不能俯仰也，求其斷接之能，非見隱顯微不可，
隱微似斷未斷，見顯似接未接，接接斷斷，斷斷接接，
其意心身體神氣，極于隱顯，又何慮不粘、黏、連、隨
哉！

When you are sparring with your opponent, you must always be cautious of the problems of bending forward and leaning backward. This means to keep your center, balance, and a firm root. The key to avoiding this is to keep your Jin and mind connected as much as possible. In addition, you should keep your spirit and alertness at a high level. When this happens, you may avoid the problem of bending forward and leaning backward.

However, occasionally you need to bend forward or lean backward to execute your techniques effectively. In this case, you must first master your skills of breaking and reconnecting. Without these skills, you will put yourself in a disadvantageous position. To reach this capability, you must learn how to conserve your Jin. Jin should not be emitted completely. Somehow, it seems the Jin is emitted yet also seems controlled. It seems controlled, yet is already emitted. In order to reach this level, you must learn the skills of storing Jin and emitting Jin from expanding postures first (i.e., large circle) and then gradually become more compact (i.e., small circle or short range). The more compactly you can execute your techniques, the easier it will be for you to reconnect when broken.

In conclusion, to avoid the problems generated from bending forward and leaning backward, you must know how to break and reconnect the Jin. To reach the capability of breaking and reconnecting, you must be able to manifest your Yi (i.e., wisdom mind), Xin (i.e., emotional mind), body, spirit, and Qi to their extreme level. When this happens, you are in a high place of awareness and alertness. This will provide good conditions to execute your skills of attaching, adhering, connecting, and following.

太
極
節
、
拿
、
抓
、
閉

、
尺
、
寸
、
分
、
毫
辨

3.31 The Discrimination of Taiji's Controlling, Seizing, Grabbing, and Sealing with Meter, Decimeter, Centimeter, and Millimeter

Once (you) have achieved the Gong (i.e., Gongfu) of sparring, then (you) can gauge (how) to apply the foot, inch, centimeter, and millimeter (Jins) at the hands. However, it does not matter how easily the techniques of controlling, seizing, grabbing, and sealing can be obtained, if (applying them in) controlling the fasciae, seizing the vessels, grabbing the tendons, and sealing the cavities, then it is difficult. If not gauged from the foot, inch, centimeter, and millimeter (Jins), they cannot be obtained. (If) controlling cannot be gauged (i.e., applied yet), then (you may) use the An (i.e., pressing down) to gain the fasciae. (If) seizing cannot be gauged (i.e., applied yet), then (you may) use the Mo (i.e., rubbing) to gain the vessels. (If) grabbing cannot be gauged (i.e., applied yet), then (you may use) the Tui (i.e., pushing) to achieve (the goal of) grabbing (the tendons). To achieve (the goal) of sealing the cavities with sealing, (you must) gauge from the feel and shorten into inch, centimeter, and millimeter. Even if these four skills have been taught by a highly proficient (master), however, without spending Gongfu by yourself for a long period of time, (you) still cannot understanding them thoroughly.

對待之功既得，尺寸分毫于手，則可以量之矣。然不論
節、拿、抓、閉之手易，若節膜、拿脈、抓筋、閉穴則
難，非自尺寸分毫量之，不可得也。節不量由按而得膜，
拿不量由摩而得脈，抓不量由推而得拿，閉非量而不能
得穴，由尺盈而縮之寸分毫也。此四者雖有高授，然非
自己功夫久者，無能貫通焉。

To reach a general level of Taijiquan sparring skill is not difficult. As long as you understand the Taijiquan fighting concepts and theories, through intelligent practice and a correct guidance from your teacher, you can reach a good level of fighting skills. From this achievement, you could also easily grasp the skills of controlling (Jie, 節), seizing (Na, 拿), grabbing (Zhua, 抓), and sealing (Bi, 閉). However, these skills remain on the general level. To reach a proficient level where the same skills can be applied in controlling the fasciae (Jie Mo, 節膜), seizing the vessels (Na Mai, 拿脈), grabbing the tendons (Zhua Jin, 抓筋), and sealing the cavities (Bi Xue, 閉穴), you must learn how to shorten your fighting range to be more compact and also more finely resolve your feeling of sensitivity from meters to decimeters, centimeters, and then to millimeters. Without this sense of feeling, you will not be able to direct your Jins to the fasciae, vessels, tendons, and cavities to make them effective.

The trick to reaching a high level of sensitive feeling is through the development of these skills: pressing downward (An, 按), scouring (Mo, 摩), and pushing (Tui, 推). With the assistance of pressing downward, you can feel the fasciae and control them; with the assistance of scouring, your feeling can reach the vessels and locate them; with the assistance of pushing, you can reach the tendons and grab them and therefore seize the opponent. Sealing the cavities is the most difficult skill which must be obtained from the training of high sensitivity and the accuracy of Jins.

However, even though the theories and concepts are easily understood and can be taught by a proficient master, it will still take great effort and practice (i.e., Gongfu, 功夫) to reach the final goal.

太極補助氣力解

3.32 The Interpretation of Nourishing and Releasing the Qi and Li in Taiji

To nourish and to release the Qi and Li to yourself is difficult. To nourish and to release the Qi and Li to the opponent is also difficult. To nourish yourself is (when you) feel there is a deficiency, then nourish it. (When) there is a sufficiency in (your) exercises (i.e., actions), then release it. Therefore, (you can see that) it is not easy to ask yourself to (reach) these (goals). To nourish the opponent is (when his) Qi is excessive then nourish (with my Qi); (when his) Li is overpowered, then release it. This is the reason why I win and the opponent loses. When Qi is excessive, then release and when the Li is overpowered, then nourish it. Though the theory remains the same, there is a detailed explanation necessary. Too much of nourishing means to add excess over excess. When encountering (opponent's) releasing, (I) further retard (his) deficiency. (When this happens,) he will over react by compensating too much and become excessive. The method of either nourishing the Qi or releasing Li to the opponent, both cause the opponent to react excessively. Nourishing Qi is called "congeal the Qi method," while releasing the Li is called "emptying the Li method."

補瀉氣力于自己難，補瀉氣力于人亦難。補自己者，知
覺功虧則補，運動功過則瀉，所以求諸己不易也。補于
人者，氣過則補之，力過則瀉之，此勝彼敗，所由然也。
氣過或瀉，力過或補，其理雖一，然其有詳。夫過補為
之過上加過，遇瀉為之緩，他不及他必更過，仍加過也。
補氣瀉力，于人之法，均為加過于人矣。補氣名曰結氣
法，瀉力名曰空力法。

Without correct understanding and intelligent practice, it is not easy to build up strong Qi within yourself and manifest it into physical actions. Jin in Chinese means "Qi" (氣) and "Li" (力). That means when Qi is manifested externally into a physical form, it is Jin.

In order to establish a high level of Jin manifestation, you must first learn how to build up your Qi in the Lower Dan Tian (Xia Dan Tian, 下丹田) and then learn how to use the concentrated mind to lead the Qi to the physical body for action. Naturally, this is not an easy task for a Taijiquan beginner. When the proper amount of Qi is led by the mind to manifest Jin, the power will be adequate for action. However, when the mind is overacting or underacting, the Qi will be either excessive or deficient. When this happens, the Jin manifested will be either too weak or too strong (i.e., overemphasized), which can be used by the opponent. The level of the mind in the action depends on the sensitivity of your feeling. Feeling is the language between your body and your mind. When your feeling is sensitive, the communication between your body and mind will be clear. This lets you direct your Qi correctly and accurately for your actions.

Only after you can build up your own Qi and manifest it externally are you able to apply it to the opponent. The ability to use your mind to manifest your Jin to the opponent's body depends on the sensitivity of your feeling (i.e., Listening Jin, 聽勁) between you and your opponent. Through this feeling, you will know if the opponent's Qi and Li is excessive or deficient so you can take advantage of it. That means you may use your Qi and Li to affect the opponent's Qi and Li. Naturally, this is also no easy task.

Strategically, when the opponent's Qi is too sufficient, then you should offer him more to overflow his Qi. However, when the opponent's Li (i.e., Qi's manifestation) has been over-manifested, then you will lead this Li into emptiness. Naturally, you may also use other strategies, such as if the opponent's Qi is too abundant (saturated), then you lead it away and when his Li is overpowered, then you add more power to it. When this happens, in order to save the situation, the opponent will often overreact and still end up with too much Qi flow and Li manifestation. From this, you can see that insubstantial and substantial actions are exchangeable, depending on how you play them. The way of nourishing the opponent's increased Qi to make it more sufficient is called "congeal the Qi method," while releasing the Li is called "emptying the Li method."

太
極
空
、
結
、
挫
、
揉
解

3.33 The Interpretation of Emptiness, Congealment, Filing, and Rubbing in Taiji

There is a distinction between filing emptiness and filing congealment; also between rubbing emptiness and rubbing congealment. (If) filing emptiness, then the Li is cornered (i.e., dull); (if) filing congealment, then the Qi is broken (i.e., without circulation); (when) rubbing emptiness, then the Qi is divided (i.e., weakened); (when) rubbing the congealment, then the Qi is cornered (i.e., stagnant). If there is a congealment, the rubbing and breaking will cause the Qi and Li to reverse. (If) there is an emptiness, the rubbing and filing will cause the Qi and Li to be defeated (i.e., weakened). If there is a congealment, the rubbing and filing will make the Li stronger than Qi, therefore Li is more than Qi. If there is an emptiness, filing and rubbing will make the Qi more excessive than Li, therefore, the Qi will be too abundant and the Li will be deficient. Whether filing (to cause) congealment or rubbing (to cause emptiness); or rubbing (to cause) congealment or filing (to cause emptiness), the Qi is sealed off due to Li. Rubbing (to cause) emptiness or breaking (to cause congealment), all because the Li is drilled (i.e., weakened) by Qi. In conclusion, the techniques of filing congealment and rubbing emptiness must also be obtained from the gauging of feet, inch, centimeter, and millimeter. Otherwise, how can (you) achieve the filing and rubbing without the root and subtle congealment without clear accuracy.

有挫空、挫結，有揉空、揉結之辨。挫空者，則力隔矣；
挫結者，則氣斷矣；揉空者，則氣分矣；揉結者，則氣
隔矣。若結，揉挫則氣力反。空，揉挫則氣力敗。結，
揉挫則力盛于氣，力在氣上矣。空，挫揉則氣盛于力，
氣過力不及矣。挫結揉，揉結挫，皆氣閉于力矣；揉空
挫，皆力鏨于氣矣。總之，挫結、揉空之法，亦必由尺
寸分毫，量能如是也。不然無地之挫揉，平虛之靈結，
亦何由而致于哉！

Filing (Cuo, 挫 and circular rubbing (Rou, 柔、揉) are the two skills which can be used to damage the fasciae and Qi vessels. Emptiness (Kong, 空)(i.e., void) and congealment (Jie, 結)(i.e., stagnation) are the consequences which can result from applications of filing and circular rubbing. When you use filing or circular rubbing techniques, it can cause either emptiness or congealment of the Qi and/or blood circulation in the struck area. There are four possible consequences when applying these two techniques: filing to cause emptiness, filing to cause congealment, circular rubbing to cause emptiness, and circular rubbing to cause congealment.

It is told that victims of emptiness caused from filing will suffer a dullness of the Li; after congealment resulting from filing, Qi circulation will be cut off. In addition, victims of emptiness caused from rubbing will suffer division of the Qi, and its misdirection to the wrong path; after congealment caused from circular rubbing, Qi circulation will be stagnant. If already congealed, the applications of rubbing and filing will cause the Qi and Li to reverse their normal condition and make the Li overreact. However, if already empty, the applications of rubbing and filing will weaken the Qi and Li and make the Qi's circulation too abundant. In addition, all of these techniques—either using filing to attack the congealment or using rubbing to attack the emptiness, or using rubbing to attack the congealment and filing to attack the emptiness—will seal the Qi circulation due to stagnation of the Li's manifestation. Other consequences, such as using rubbing to attack the emptiness or filing the congealment, etc. will make the Li weaken from the influence of the Qi.

In my personal opinion, I really wonder if there is still any martial artist who has reached such a high level of martial skill today. To achieve this goal, it would take a lifetime of intelligent practice with correct guidance. It is almost impossible to reach this level in today's world.

懂
勁
先
後
論

3.34 The Thesis of Before and After Understanding Jin

Before gaining the ability of Understanding Jin, (we) often commit the errors of excess, deficiency, separating, and resistance. After knowing the Understanding Jin, (we) are again afraid of making the errors of breaking, connecting, bending forward, and leaning backward. It is understood that before Understanding Jin, it is easier (for us) to make errors. But how (can we) still make errors even after (we have) understood Jin? This is because when the understanding of Jin is between understood and not understood, both ways are possible, then breaking and connecting are without a standard (i.e., guideline). Therefore, the errors are made. (If) the spiritual enlightenment has not been achieved yet, bending forward and leaning backward without the root (i.e., capability of breaking and reconnecting), then errors can also be made. If (you) do not learn and exit from making errors in breaking, connecting, leaning forward, and bending backward, then (you are) not really Understanding Jin. In this case, how can (you) really Understand Jin if (you) do not have the essential (training of your) vision and hearing (i.e., feeling), thus, the accuracy cannot be obtained.

夫未懂勁之先，長出頂、匾、丟、抗之病；既懂勁之後，恐出斷、接、俯、仰之病。然未懂勁故然病亦出勁，既懂何以出病乎？緣勁似懂未懂之際，正在兩可，斷接無準矣，故出病。神明及猶不及，俯仰無著矣，亦出病。若不出斷、接、俯、仰之病，非真懂勁，弗能不出也。胡為真懂？因視聽無由，未得其確也。

Before understanding Jin, you always make errors of its excess or deficiency, as well as separating and resistance (i.e., double weighting) during contact with your opponent. Even if you understand the generalized application of Jin, you will still commit the mistakes of broken and reconnected Jin, and also the problem of bending forward or leaning backward. The reason for this is simply because you are in the stage between "not understanding" and "understanding." However, making mistakes is the correct path to reaching more deep and profound levels of Understanding Jin. Only if you reach to a level of spiritual enlightenment (i.e., high level of alertness and awareness) can you then bend forward and lean backward without any problem. It is only then that you will be able to break and reconnect easily. The way of reaching a higher, more enlightened level of Understanding Jin is to train your feeling sensitivity (i.e., listening) and alertness (i.e., eyes' vision or awareness).

(If your) vision is able to know far and near, left and right; (your) hearing is able to perceive the rising, falling, slow, and fast; (you) are familiar with the actions of dodging, returning, provoking, and ceasing; and (you) can feel the movements of turning, exchanging, advancing, and retreating, then you have really (reached the level of) Understanding Jin. (When this happens,) then are (you) able to reach the spiritual enlightenment, and thus all of the spirit's to and fro have their reasons. When there is a reason, it is because of Understanding Jin. Consequently, (you) will acquire the marvelousness of the bending, extending, moving, and stillness. When there is a marvelousness of bending, extending, moving, and stillness, then opening, closing, rising, and falling again have their reasons (of actions). Based on bending, extending, moving, and stillness; when seeing entering, then open; when encountering (i.e., contacting), then close; when seeing coming, then fall; when seeing going, then rise. Only then it is clear that (you) have really reached the spiritual enlightenment. (After reaching this level,) how can (you) not be cautious in (your) walking, sitting, lying down, diet, and elimination. This is how (you) reach the middle and great achievements.

知瞻眇顧盼之視，覺起落緩急之聽，知閃還撩了之運，
覺轉換進退之動，則為真懂勁，則能接及神明，及神明
自攸往有由矣。有由者，由于懂勁，自得屈伸動靜之妙。
有屈伸動靜之妙，開合升降，又有由矣。由屈伸動靜，
見入則開，遇之則合，看來則降，就去則升，夫而後才
為真及神明也明也。豈可日後不慎行坐臥走，飲食溺溷
之功，是所為及中成、大成也哉！

Your level of alertness and awareness depends on the refinement of your senses—chiefly from the eyes' contact, the ears' listening, and the skin's feeling when touched. When you have high alertness and awareness, you can know far and near, left and right; you can perceive the rising, falling, slowness, and swiftness; you become familiar with the maneuvers of dodging, returning, provoking, and ceasing; and you can enact the movements of turning, exchanging, advancing, and retreating clearly. This is really the state of Understanding Jin.

Only after you are familiar with Understanding Jin can your judgments, decisions, and actions be clear and accurate. This is the path of reaching spiritual enlightenment. Once your spirit is able to control the entire combat situation, you will have not only high morale and alertness, but also precise action. In this case, you know your opponent's action and your reaction without any doubt. During the process of this refinement, first you acquire the skills of bending, extending, moving, and stillness, then opening, closing, rising, and falling. From these acquisitions, you can open and close with advantageous timing and tactics.

To reach this enlightened level of Taijiquan is a long and trying training process. Once you have reached this level, how can you not be but cautious about your life? If you risk your life easily, you have wasted all of the efforts. You chose the moment.

3.35 The Thesis of Meter, Decimeter, Centimeter, and Millimeter after Understanding Jin

Before (knowing) Understanding Jin, if (you) first search for (the skills of) meter, decimeter, centimeter, and millimeter (Jins), (even they are accomplished,) it is still considered little achievement since they are only the superficial level of martial arts (skills). Whoever can apply the foot Jin to the opponent, does not necessary have to know the Understanding Jin first. (However,) if (you) have (mastered) the Understanding Jin already, (your) spirit will have been enlightened (i.e., understood the opponent's intention). (In this case,) naturally, (you) can gauge the foot and inch (Jins). (Only) when the foot and inch Jins can be gauged, can (you) control, seize, grab, and seal. In order to know the theory of (applying techniques to) fasciae, vessels, tendons, and cavities, (you) must know (the skills) of the life and death hands' (vital skills) clearly. In order to know the hands' (vital skills) of life and death, (you) must know the cavities of life and death clearly. How can (you) not know the number of cavities (which can be used)? (Once you) know the number of the life and death cavities, how can (you) not know (those cavities) can be sealed and not alive (i.e., killed)? How can (you) not know (those cavities which) can be sealed and not alive (i.e., killed)? (repetition in original document) What is called the life and death two words, completely depends on the sole (technique) of sealing.

在懂勁先求尺寸分毫，為之小成，不過末技武事而已。所謂能尺于人者，非先懂勁也。如懂勁後，神而明之，自然能量尺寸。尺寸能量，才能節、拿、抓、閉矣。知膜脈筋穴之理，要必明存亡之手。知存亡之手，要必明生死之穴。其穴之數，安可不知乎？知生死之穴數，烏可不明閉而不生乎？烏可不明閉而不生乎？是所謂二字之存亡，一閉之而已盡矣。

尺、寸、分、毫在懂勁後論

If you do not know Understanding Jin, even if you have figured out the distance for each Jin's manifestation, what you can achieve is still on the superficial level of martial accomplishment. To reach a proficient level of martial skill, you must know Understanding Jin. Understanding Jin can be acquired from the training of alertness and awareness. In order to reach a high level of alertness and awareness, you must first build up a high level of sensory sensitivity. The more sensitive your feeling, the shorter the Jin you can execute. When this happens, you can use the skills of controlling the fasciae, seizing the vessels, grabbing the tendons, and sealing the cavities. Naturally, in order to make these techniques effective, you must know how many places and exactly where they are in order to execute your techniques effectively. According to martial arts training, out of the more than 700 acupuncture cavities, there are 108 cavities which can be used for martial arts or for healing massage. Among these 108 cavities, 72 are not vital while the other 36 can cause death when struck with precisely correct power and timing. Normally, the locations and the effective timings of these cavities were kept secret until a master was able to trust the student completely. In addition, the special training to make the attack effective was also commonly kept secret.

3.36 The Explanation of Taijiquan's Fingers, Palms, and Pounding Hands

The internal area from the base of the fingers to the wrist is the palm. (Together with) five leading fingers is called hand. All five fingers are individual. When holding the five fingers, the back side is called a fist. In applications, press down (i.e., An) and push (i.e., Tui) use the palm. Seizing, rubbing, grabbing, and sealing all use fingers. Filing and scouring use hands. Punch uses fist. About punches, there are "deflect downward and parry," "aim for crotch," "under the elbow," and "turning the body." Other than these four punches, there is "reversed fist." About palms (techniques), there are "brush the knee," "exchange and turn," "single whip," "fan back." Other than these four palms applications, there is "thread palm." About the hands (techniques), there are "cloud hands," "lift hand," "grab," and "cross hands." Other than these four hands (techniques), there is a "reverse hand." About the fingers (finger applications), there are "bent finger," "extended fingers," "pinch finger," and "sealing finger." Other than these four fingers (finger applications), there is a "measuring (or gauging) finger," which is also named "foot and inch finger," or "seeking for cavity finger."

太極指掌捶手解

自指下之腕上，裡者為掌，五指之首為之手，五指皆為指，五指權里其背為捶。如其用者，按、推，掌也；拿、揉、抓、閉，俱用指也；挫、摩，手也；打，捶也。夫捶有搬攔，有指襠，有肘底，有撇身，四捶之外有覆捶；掌有摟膝，有換轉，有單鞭，有通背，四掌之外有串掌；手有雲手，有提手，拿，有十字手，四手之外有反手；指有屈指，有伸指，捏指，閉指，四指之外有量指，又名尺寸指，又名覓穴指。

This paragraph explains the structure of the hand and also what techniques can be used from different parts of the hands. In addition, it also gives many examples of the explanation for the names of the Taijiquan forms.

However, there are five fingers and each of these five fingers has its applications. Though they are connected (with the palm) as a hand, their functions remain as fingers. Therefore, they are also named "hand-fingers." Its first applications are "rotating fingers," and "rotating hand." Its second applications are "root fingers," and "root hand." Its third applications are "bow fingers," and "bow hand." Its fourth applications are "central unification," and "hand fingers." Other than these four fingers, there are "single finger," and "single hand." Index finger is "urgent finger," "sword finger," "assistant finger," and "adhering finger." The middle finger is "heart finger," "unification finger," "hooking finger," and "smearing finger." The ring finger is "complete finger," "ring finger," "substitute finger," and "plucking finger." The little finger is "aiding finger," "mending finger," "seductive finger," and "hanging finger." It is easy to know these terminologies but difficult to apply them. Even if (you) have obtained the oral secret, it is still not easy (to apply them).

然指有五指，有五指之用，首指為手仍為指，故又名手指，其一用之為旋指、旋手，其二用之為根指，根手，其三用之為弓指、弓手，其四用之為中合、手指。四手指之外為獨指，獨手也。食指為卞指，為劍指，為佐指，為粘指；中指為心指，為合指，為鉤指，為抹指；無名指為全指，為環指，為代指，為扣指；小指為幫指，補指，媚指，掛指。若此之名，知之易而用之難，得口訣秘法，亦不易為也。

This paragraph explains the applications of each finger. Many of the names mentioned were created and used in different martial styles. Therefore, in order to obtain their secrets of use, personal instruction from a master in the style is necessary.

Then, there are "matching palms," "pushing the mountain palm," "shooting the goose palm," "spreading the wings palm," "as close as seal finger," "twist stepping finger," "bend the bow finger," "threading the shuttle finger," "patting the horse hand," "bending the bow hand," "embracing the tiger hand," "jade lady hand," "riding the tiger hand," "through the mountain punch," "under the leaf punch," "reversed punch," "separating the posture punch," "wrapping filing punch." (In addition, you must) change (your) stepping following the body's maneuver, without being apart from (the theory of) Five Elements; then there is no mistake. This is because (if you have understood) the theory of attaching, connecting, adhering, and following, giving up yourself and following the opponent, the body follows and the stepping automatically changes. As long as there is no mistake in applying Five Elements, the body and the stepping are natural, then how (do you) worry about some little mistakes that have been done.

其次有對掌、推山掌、射雁掌、晾翅掌、似閉指、拗步指、彎弓指、穿梭指、探馬手、彎弓手、抱虎手、玉女手、跨虎手、通山捶、葉下捶、背反捶、勢分捶、卷挫捶，再其次步隨身換，不出五行，則無失錯矣。因其粘、連、黏、隨之理，舍己從人，身隨步自換，只要無五行之舛錯，身形腳勢出于自然，又何慮些須之病也。

Again, this paragraph explains the uses of the palms and hands. The techniques or the movements of each name must be instructed by the master individually.

In addition, this paragraph also mentions that in order to make all the techniques effective, you must master the maneuvers of Five Steppings (Wu Bu, 五步). The stepping and the body's action follow, coordinate, and harmonize with each other. Only then can you execute the skills of attaching, connecting, adhering, and following effectively.

3.37. The Thesis of Oral Transmission of Life and Death in Cavities

The cavities include those cavities (which, when attacked) can remain alive or cause death. (However), they must be taught orally. Why? One, because it is hard to learn; two, because it is related to life and death; three, because it depends on the personal learning talent. First, do not teach to those who are not loyal and filial. Second, do not teach to those who do not have a good (martial) foundation. Third, do not teach to those whose hearts (i.e., mind) are not righteous (i.e., evil). Fourth, do not teach to those who are rude and careless. Fifth, do not teach to those who are too proud of themselves and do not respect others. Six, do not teach to those who know the politeness but without benevolence. Seventh, do not teach to those who change their mind all the time (i.e., cannot be trusted). Eighth, do not teach to those who obtain easily and also lose easily (i.e., do not appreciate deeply). These are the eight (kinds of people who) cannot be taught; do not even mention teaching to those outlaws. If a person can be taught, then teach him the secrets orally. Pass to those who know loyalty, filial piety, and appreciation; to those whose heart (i.e., mind) and Qi are harmonious and peaceful; to those who could keep the Dao without losing it; to those who can really treat a teacher as a teacher; to those who can last from the beginning until the end. If a person is able to last from the beginning until the end, without changing (his mind) and maintaining (his) original (thinking)(i.e., be consistent), then it is obvious that (you) should teach him the total great applications. (These rules) are the same in the past and also in the future, pass them down generation by generation all should follow as such. Alas! Don't (you) know that there are many gangsters in martial society.

口授穴之存亡論

穴有存亡之穴，要非口授不可。何也？一因難學，二因
關系存亡，三因其人才能傳。第一不授不忠不孝之人，
第二不傳根底不好之人，第三不授心術不正之人，第四
不傳鹵莽滅裂之人，第五不傳授目中無人之人，第六不
傳知禮無恩之人，第七不授反復無長（常）之人，第八
不傳得易失易之人。此須知八不傳，匪人更不待言矣。
如其可以傳，再口授之秘訣。傳忠孝知恩者，心氣和平
者，守道不失者，真以為師者，始終如一者。果其有始
有終，不變如一，方可將全體大用之功，授之于徒也明
矣。于前于後，代代相繼，皆如是之所傳也。噫！抑亦
知武事中烏有匪人哉！

Pressing cavity (Dian Xue, 點穴), sealing the vessel (Duan Mai, 斷脈), controlling the fasciae (Jie Mo, 節膜), and grabbing the tendons (Zhua Jin, 抓筋) are the four higher levels of martial skills. Among these four, pressing cavity and sealing the vessel can cause death when used. Therefore, a traditional master will not teach these skills to a student easily. This paragraph lists eight kinds of students to whom a master should not pass down these skills and secrets. Only this can prevent these skills from being used by bad people and causing problems to society.

3.38 The Legacy of Zhang, San-Feng

Heaven and earth are Qian and Kun, Fu Xi is the ancestor of mankind. (Who) drew (i.e., created) the trigram and (therefore) the Dao had the name, (which descended down) to Yao, Shun, and sixteen mothers (i.e., generations). Allowed to keep the center (i.e., balance or truth) cautiously, (its) sole refinement (i.e., pure Dao) had passed down to Confucius and Mencius. The Gongfu of spiritual cultivation in both human life and human nature, has been exemplified in seventy-two (generations) until (the Han emperors of) Wen and Wu. This teaching has been passed down to us through (a person) named Xu, Xuan-Ping. The herb (i.e., elixir) of extending life is in the body, (from it) the original goodness will be repeated from the beginning. Insubstantial supernatural spirit is able to make the human virtue bright, (when) regulated (correctly), the Qi and the shape (i.e., physical body) can be completed in whole. For ten thousand years, (we can) chant (and praise) the long spring (i.e., eternal youth), the sincere heart (i.e., the mind) could keep the truthful relics. (The Dao) of teaching from three schools do not have two families (i.e., no difference), all what they talk about is Taiji. Its greatness has filled (the universe) strongly. It has set up the rules which will last for thousands of years. (We should) follow and continue the ancient sages' teaching and make it last forever. (We should also) always open our mind to allow the newcomers to continue this task. Once the water (i.e., Yin) and fire (i.e., Yang) can support each other mutually (i.e., be harmonious with each other), it is wished to last until the end of our lives.

張三豐承留

天地即乾坤，伏羲為人祖。畫卦道有名，堯舜十六母。
微危允厥中，精一及孔孟。神化性命功，七二及文武。
授之至予來，字著宣平許。延年藥在身，元善從復始。
虛靈能德明，理令氣形具。萬載詠長春，心分誠真跡。
三教無兩家，統言皆太極。浩然塞而沖，方正千年立。
繼往聖永綿，開來學常續。水火濟既焉，願至戍畢字。

Nature is commonly referred to as "heaven and earth" by the Chinese. The heavens are considered Qian (乾) while the earth is Kun (坤) in the Eight Trigrams. It was believed that the concept and theories of Taiji and the Eight Trigrams were created by Fu Xi (伏羲) (2852-2737 B.C.), the ancestor of the Chinese Han race. From these concepts and the theories, the Chinese were able to follow the natural Qi balance and all prosperity was derived. This philosophy was finally passed down to Xu, Xuan-Ping (許宣平) who is believed to have been one of the possible creators or pioneers of Taijiquan. From practicing Taijiquan, you can maintain your physical, living health and raise up your spirit to cultivate your natural potential as a human being. The three schools (San Jiao, 三教) are Buddhism, Daoism, and Confucianism. All of these schools have followed the philosophy of Taiji and the Eight Trigrams, and from the study of this philosophy, they can understand the great Qi and spirit of nature, and its truth and righteousness. After we have learned Taijiquan, we should continue this study and development to understand the balance of Yin (i.e., water) and Yang (i.e., fire). In this case, the Dao of Taiji and the concept of Yin and Yang can be passed down to many generations to come.

3.39 The Oral Transmission of Zhang, San-Feng's Lecture

We know that the theory (of the Dao) belongs as one (i.e., is the same) in all three educational schools (i.e., Buddhist, Daoist, and Confucian). They all study the physical life and human nature and all consider the mind (i.e., Xin) is the master of the body. When the mind and the physical body are protected safely (i.e., healthily), then (you) will have Jing (i.e., essence), Qi, and Shen (i.e., spirit) forever. If (you) have Jing, Qi, and Shen, then are (you) able to cultivate the mental mind peacefully and maintain the martial activities active (i.e., physical exercise). Keeping peaceful (mental mind) and (martial) activities, then (you) have acquired the scholarship (i.e., mentality, internal understanding) and martial capability (i.e., physical strength or actions). Those who have reached (to) a great level, become sagehood and deity (i.e., immortality). Those who have (been) enlightened (in these studies) before others, can keep the human virtue in the ring (i.e., comprehend the meaning of life) and understand beyond the physical appearance. Those who have comprehended later, must model (i.e., follow) the knowledge and capabilities of those who have (become) enlightened earlier. Though this knowledge and capability are the natural innate capability for all of us, however, they cannot be acquired without being educated. This is because we have the natural born capabilities in mentality (i.e., mental understanding) and martial activities (i.e., physical exercises). The eyes can see, the ears can hear are the natural capabilities of scholarship. The hands dancing and the feet stepping are the natural capabilities of martial activities. Therefore, it is clear that (we) all have these capabilities.

口授張三豐老師之言

予知三教歸一之理，皆性命學也，皆以心為身之主也，
保全心身，永有精氣神也。有精氣神，才能文思安安，
武備動動，安安動動，乃文乃武，大而化之者，聖神也。
先覺者，德其衷中，超乎象外矣；後覺者，以效先覺之
所知能，其知能雖人固有之知能，然非效之不可得也。
夫人之知能，天然文武。目視耳聽，天然文也，手舞足
蹈，天然武也，孰非固有也明矣。

The three educational schools are: Buddhism, Daoism, and Confucianism. These three schools are the most influential groups that have long dominated Chinese thinking and philosophy. Each of these three schools focuses on the philosophical development of human nature (i.e., internal mental cultivation) through comprehension and physical health through physical activities (i.e., martial activities). Moreover, each of these schools believes that the mind is the master of the entire being, and controls our thinking and physical activities. In order to reach the goal of mental or spiritual cultivation and physical health, you must know how to protect and firm your essence (Gu Jing, 固精), nourish your Qi (Yang Qi, 養氣), and raise up your spirit (Ti Shen, 提神). These three things are considered the three treasures of life (San Bao, 三寶). Only if you know how to do these things are you able to have a peaceful, calm, and profound mind to think, ponder, and understand. Moreover, you will be able to perform your physical activities healthily.

Those who can comprehend the Dao internally and apply it into external, physical actions with a great level of achievement will reach spiritual enlightenment and sagehood. Those who have a high awareness and can understand the Dao and manifest it externally will become the pioneers of human internal and external cultivation. Finally, those who do not have a high level of comprehension and awareness will have to learn from those who do understand. From this, you can see that although all humans have eyes, ears, a brain, hands, and feet, the difference still can be so great.

(Our) ancestors who have reached the great achievement in both scholarly (i.e., internal spiritual) and martial (i.e., external physical) cultivation(s) taught us how

to use exercise (i.e., physical movements) to cultivate (our) physical body, and advance (into the stage of) not (just) using the martial arts to cultivate (our body). After passing down to us, (we) can acquire the essence of battle (i.e., essential movements learned from combat) in the hands' movements and the feet's stepping, which (allows us to) borrow the body's Yin to nourish the body's Yang. The body's Yang is male while the body's Yin is female, all existing in our body. A male's body is all Yin but a place is Yang. Female absorbs this sole Yang to battle the entire body's Yin. Therefore, it is said, the female is repeating from the beginning due to sole Yang. When (we) talk about Yin in (our) body, it is not only female who possesses seven-two (i.e., post-pubescent essence). Using the name (i.e., method) of "fair lady" to match "baby boy" is able to transform into millions of variations. Therefore, a "fair lady" is able to pick up the essence as well. There are also some males or females who use the post-birth bodies to nourish themselves. This is what is called to use the self's heaven and earth (i.e., Yin and Yang) to assist the self. This is the method of picking up the essence of Yin and Yang to nourish each other. This is the case for a male that the entire body belongs to Yin and use the self Yin to battle the self female. In this kind of cultivation, the accomplishment is not as rapid as two males' mutual Yin and Yang nourishment.

前輩大成文武聖神，授人以體育修身，進之不以武事修身，傳之至予，得之手舞足蹈之采戰，借其身之陰，以補助身之陽。身之陽男也，身之陰女也，然皆于身中矣。男之身只一陽，男全身皆陰，女以一陽采戰全體之陰，女故云一陽復始。斯身之陰，女不獨七二，以一妊女配嬰兒之名，變化千萬，妊女采戰之可也。亦安有男女後天之身以補之者，所謂自身之天地以扶助之，是為陰陽采戰也。如此者，是男子之身皆屬陰，而采自身之陰，戰己身之女，不如兩男之陰陽對待，修身速也。

Internal understanding is Yin while external physical manifestation is Yang. At the beginning, we learn how to move our body naturally. This is a natural pre-born capability. After we have moved for a long time, we start to ponder internally and try to understand the movements and make them more efficient and powerful. Therefore, we are using Yin (i.e., internal understanding) to nourish our Yang.

In analyzing the human body, there are again classifications of Yang and Yin. Yang is considered male while Yin is considered female. Therefore, within your body, there are both male (Yang) and female (Yin) that can be used to nourish, harmonize, and support each other. This theory can also be applied to two persons, one male and one female. From a Qigong perspective, though a male's physical body is Yang, however, his Qi body is Yin; conversely, while a female's physical body is Yin, her Qi body is Yang. Although a male's entire Qi body is Yin, there is a place where the Qi is extremely Yang. This place is the penis, which is used to balance the entire body's Yin. Although a female's physical body is Yin, she can obtain the male's Yang and turn herself into stronger Yang. When this happens, due to the interaction of Yin and Yang, a new life is derived.

When we talk about Yin in a body, it is not only the female who possesses post-pubescent essence (i.e., seven-two possibly implies fourteen years of age). When a young lady (Cha Nu, 姹女) is coupled with a young boy (Ying Er, 嬰兒)(i.e., Yin and Yang interaction), millions of variations can be derived.

However, you must also understand that Yin and Yang mutual nourishment is not limited to one male and one female. In fact, often it is believed in Daoist society that two males and two females can also nourish each other. This kind of practice is called "double cultivation" (Shuang Xiu, 雙修). It is said in Daoist society: "Yin and Yang are not necessarily male and female, the strength and the weakness of Qi in the body are Yin and Yang."[8] It is again said: "Two men can plant and graft and a pair of women can absorb and nourish."[9]

I have applied these (methods) to martial arts, however, (you) must not view them as superficial skills. They

*remain as a study of physical exercises, the Dao of cul-
tivating the body and human nature, and the realm of
reaching sagehood and the divine. Now, the battle of
absorbing essence between two males and the battle of
absorbing essence within ourselves have no difference in
theory. When we encounter the correct number (i.e.,
matching, Yin-Yang interaction), then it is the battle of
adopting essence. It is the process of mercury and lead.
When we encounter an opponent in a battle, the Yin
and Yang of Kan, Li, Dui, and Zhen in the trigrams
perform the way of Yang seizing Yin, and is the four
directions (in Taijiquan). The Yin and Yang of Qian,
Kun, Gen, and Xun, demonstrate the way of Yin adopting Yang, and is the four corners (in Taijiquan). This is
the Eight Trigrams and is "eight doors" (in action). The
body and feet are located in the central earth. When we
advance, we use Yang to seize the opponent; when we
retreat, we use Yin to adopt the opponent; when we pay
attention to the left, we use Yang to adopt the opponent;
and when we look to the right, we use Yin to seize the
opponent. This is the Five Phases and is "five steppings"
(in action). Total there are "eight doors and five steppings." What I have just instructed you can be used for
your lifetime without exhausting it. As I obtained (i.e.,
learned) martial arts, I continue my martial arts (without stop). Therefore, (I) must also pass down these martial arts (to the next generation) for body's cultivation.
When self-cultivation has been listed as the first priori-
ty, then it does not matter whether it can be achieved
from martial arts or internal spiritual, it can succeed.
The origin of the three schools' teaching and the three
levels of achievement is nothing else but Taiji. I wish
those students in the future could use the principles of
Yi Jing and apply it in their bodies, then (they can) pass
it down to future generations.*

予及此傳于武事，然不可以末技視，依然體育之學，修
身之道，性命之功，聖神之境也。今夫兩男之對待采戰，
于己身之采戰，其理不二，己身亦遇對待之數，則為采
戰也，是為汞鉛也。于人對戰，坎離之陰陽兌震，陽戰
陰也，為之四正，乾坤之陰陽艮巽，陰采陽也，為之四
隅。此八卦也，為之八門。身足位列中土，進步之陽以
戰之，退步之陰以采之，左顧之陽以采之，右盼之陰以
戰之，此五行也，為之五步。共為八門五步也。夫如是，
予授之，爾終身用之不能盡之矣。又至予得武繼武，必
當以武事傳之而修身也。修身入首，無論武事文，為成
功一也。三教三乘之原，不出一太極。願後學以易理格
致于身中，留于後世可也。

The philosophy of Taiji, Yin-Yang, and Bagua (Eight Trigrams) has been commonly applied in many aspects of Chinese life and therefore, it has existed in Chinese culture since the book *Yi Jing* (易經)(i.e., *Book of Changes*) became available. This philosophy has also been applied in Chinese martial arts. Even after its adoption into Chinese martial arts, it has remained as a philosophy for reaching the Dao in the self-cultivation of internal spirit and external physical training. When this theory is applied within our body, we are searching for the balance of Yin and Yang, and when it is applied to martial arts, we are also searching for the Yin (i.e., insubstantial) and Yang (i.e., substantial) strategies to battle an opponent. In Chinese medicine, lead is considered Yin while mercury is considered Yang. Therefore, it is common that lead and mercury are used to represent Yin and Yang.

When you apply the above theory into martial actions, then the eight trigrams will match the eight directions (i.e., eight doors, 八門). In Taijiquan, these eight directions correspond to eight basic Jin patterns. These eight Jin patterns mutually support each other and also conquer each other. When they are applied in an action coordinately and harmoniously, thousands of techniques can be derived.

In addition to these eight Jin patterns, there are also five strategic steppings or movements. These include: forward, backward, left, right, and center. These five steppings are simply called "five steppings" (Wu Bu, 五步). It is from these eight Jin patterns and five steppings that Taijiquan was created.

3.40 The Thesis of Comprehending the Dao from Martial Arts by Zhang, San-Feng

Before the creation of heaven and earth, there was a natural law first. This natural law is the control of the Qi's Yin and Yang. From the control of this natural law, heaven and earth are created and the Dao is existing within. The Dao of the Yin and Yang Qi's circulation is through interaction of these two opposite forces. These mutually interacting opposite forces are what have been defined as Yin and Yang. One Yin and one Yang means Dao. Dao does not have a name, and is the beginning of heaven and earth. When Dao can be named, it is the mother of millions of things. Before there was heaven and earth, it was a Wuji state (i.e., no extremity) and there was no name. However, after there was heaven and earth, then there are extremities, and names were given. Nevertheless, the rules before the creation of heaven and earth, is natural law (i.e., Li), after the creation of heaven and earth, is motherhood. This is the derivation of the natural law. Due to the pre-heaven's Yin-Yang and the Qi number being decided (i.e., destiny of nature), the motherhood is derived. (From this motherhood), the Post-heaven's embryo or egg is maturing in the water (i.e., womb). When the position of heaven and earth has been situated, millions of lives are raised. This is the neutral harmony of the Dao.

蓋未有天地先有理，理為氣之陰陽主宰。主宰理以有天地，道在其中。陰陽氣道之流行，則為對待。對待者，陰陽也，數也。一陰一陽之為道。道無名，天地始；道有名，萬物母。未有天地之前，無極也，無名也；既有天地之後，有極也，有名也。然前天地者曰理，後天地者曰母，是乃理化。先天陰陽氣數母生，後天胎卵溼化。位天地，育萬育，道中和然也。

There is a natural law or rule (i.e., Li, 理) that existed even before the material universe was created. From this law, the Qi's Yin and Yang have been discriminated. From Yin and Yang Qi's interactions, millions of objects and lives were derived. Therefore, a universe (i.e., heaven and earth) was created and the Dao (道)(i.e., natural way) is demonstrated within. When Yin and Yang's Qi lose their balance, the Qi will circulate and Yin and Yang will interact with each other. This interaction is therefore the way of Yin and Yang's natural behavior. The extent of this interaction depends on the extent (i.e., number, 數) of the imbalances within Yin and Yang. Through this Yin-Yang interaction, the natural force or the natural way (i.e., Dao) was formed. The Dao does not have a name, and was the beginning of the universe. However, when names were given to all of the creations, the Dao became the creator (i.e., mother) of objects and lives.

Before the material universe was created, there was a Wuji (無極) state (i.e., no extremity). Since there was nothingness, there was no name. That means the Dao had no name before the creation of the material world. When Yin and Yang Qi were discriminated, the universe (i.e., heaven and earth) was created. Since then, everything has had Yin and Yang and therefore, discrimination and naming is possible. From this, we can see that before the material world was created, the Dao was only a natural law or rule (Li, 理). After the universe was created, then the Dao itself discriminated Yin and Yang. Therefore, millions of objects were derived and the Dao became the mother of these objects. This is the variation and derivation of the Dao. Still, even after the Yin-Yang discrimination, the Dao remains neutral (i.e., truthful and balanced).

Therefore, Qian (i.e., Yang or the heaven) and Kun (i.e., Yin or the earth) are the great father and mother which were Pre-Heaven (i.e., prenatal). Our parents are the small father and mother which were Post-Heaven (i.e., postnatal). We, after obtaining the Yin and Yang's Pre-Heaven and Post-Heaven's Qi, are born with a physical body. This is the beginning of a human life. Thus, how a human being is formalized is by obtaining the great father and mother's natural life virtue which originated from the natural rule, (also) by gaining the

small father and mother's essence, blood, and skeletons.
From this combination of the Pre-Heaven and Post-
Heaven's natural virtue and life, we have become
human beings. Together with the heaven and the earth,
we become the "San Cai" (i.e., Three Powers) of nature.
In this case, how can the origin of human natural virtue
be lost. However, if (we) can keep the human nature,
then (we) will not lose our origin. If (we) do not lose
(our) original face (i.e., original human nature), then
how can we lose the direction of our physical body's
future? If (we) wish to find the place of the future (i.e.,
direction), (we) must first know where is the origin of
(our) coming. There is a door (i.e., way) to come and
there is a path to go. (In this case, we) know (ourselves)
for sure. Then, what are the ways? It is the natural
knowledge and capability that (we) were born with. It
does not matter whether we are smart or stupid, virtuous
or not, all can use this innate knowledge and capabili-
ty to approach the Dao. Since (we) can cultivate the
Dao, (we) can know where is (our) origin and also
understand where we are going. Knowing where (we)
came from and where (we will) go to, (we) can cultivate
(ourselves) to improve (our) body. Therefore, it is said
that from emperor to layman, all use self-body-cultiva-
tion as the foundation (of the Dao).

故乾坤為大父母，先天也，爹娘為小父母，後天也。得
陰陽先後天之氣，以降生身，則為人之初也。夫人身之
來者，得大父母之命性賦理，得小父母之精血形骸，合
先後天之身命，我得而成人也。以配天地為三才，安可
失性之本哉！然能率性，則本不失，既不失本來面目，
又安可失身體之去處哉！夫欲尋去處，先知來處，來有
門，去有路，良有以也。然有何以之？以之固有之知能。
無論知愚賢否，固有知能，皆可以進道。既能修道，可
知來處之源，必能去處之委。來源去委既知，能必明身
不修。故曰自天子至于庶人，壹是皆以修身為本。

When we apply this Dao into our lives, we can see that nature is
the great parent of us all, and our biological fathers and mothers are

our "small" parents. Since we were born within the great nature, our bodies are also part of nature, and manifest in their form a small heaven and earth (i.e., natural Dao). Together with heaven and earth, humanity has become one of three most powerful natural forces we currently know. San Cai (三才) means "Three Powers."

Since we are a part of nature, from understanding ourselves we can comprehend the Dao of the natural world. From training our physical body, we can make our lives healthy and long. In order to know ourselves, we must first understand the natural Dao, so that we can comprehend the way of life (i.e., where we come from and where we are going). In order to comprehend this, we must cultivate our internal wisdom and spirit. From this internal cultivation, we can manifest this internal understanding and cultivation into external actions. From these external actions, we can gain health and longevity.

But how (do we) cultivate (our) body? Use the innate knowledge and capabilities, such as the seeing of the eyes and the hearing of the ears to (increase our) wisdom and brightness (i.e., understanding). Also from the hands' movements and the stamping of the feet (i.e., physical movements), (we) will reach martial and spiritual capability. (To reach this goal, we must) pursue the very source of learning, study thoroughly, and keep our mind sincere and the intention righteous. The mind is the master of the entire body. When the mind is righteous and sincere, it can be used to stamp the feet following the Five Phases and move the hands following the Eight Trigrams. Hands and feet are Four Phases. When (they are) used (i.e., trained) with special ways, the innate capability will return to its origin. The eyes view the Three Unifications and the ears listen to the Six ways. The eyes and ears are also Four Appearances (i.e., Four Phases). Though they are situated on the surface of the body, the knowledge obtained can lead your innate knowledge back to its origin. The ears, eyes, hands, and feet can be divided into two, this is the Two Poles. All of these combine together, become a single unit and become Taiji. This is condensed from external into internal and also emitted from internal to external. If (you) are capable of doing so, then outside or inside, refined or coarse, there is no place that cannot be reached (which allows you to) comprehend (the Dao) suddenly. The wish of reaching sagehood and holiness can be achieved. To be wise and knowledgeable and to be sage and spiritual, by this is meant to complete (i.e., cultivate till the very end)(our) human nature and to establish (our) physical life. Herein, the perfection of the spirit is reached. How to reach the heaven Dao and human Dao all rely simply on sincerity.

夫修身以何？以之良知良能，視目聽耳，曰聰曰明，手
舞足蹈，乃武乃文，致知格物，意誠心正。心為一身之
主，正意誠心，以足蹈五行，手舞八卦。手足為之四象，
用之殊途，良能還原。目視三合，耳聽六道，目耳亦是
四形，體之一表，良知歸本。耳目手足，分而為二，皆
為兩儀，合之為一，共為太極，此由外斂入之于內，亦
自內發出之外也。能如是表里精粗無不到，豁然貫通，
希賢希聖之功自臻。于曰睿曰智，乃聖乃神，所謂盡性
立命，窮神達化在茲矣。然天道人道，一誠而已矣。

In this case, how do we reach the Dao through cultivation? Our eyes, ears, nose, skin feeling are the tools which allow us to contact the outside world. From this contact, our minds are touched, and through analysis and pondering, we are educated and our knowledge is increased. From this repeated and persistent information collection through our sensory organs and the mind's repeated pondering, we can reach a final internal spiritual comprehension and enlightenment. The Five Phases (Wu Xing, 五行) are: metal (Jin, 金), wood (Mu, 木), water (Shui, 水), fire (Huo, 火), and earth (Tu, 土) which correspond to the feet's steppings: forward, backward, step to left, step to right, and central equilibrium. The Three Unifications are the unification of hands and feet (Shou Jiao, 手腳), internal thinking and external action (i.e., mind and body)(Nei Wai, 內外), and the Qi's unification from the internal organs to the surface of the skin (Biao

Li, 表裡). These Three Unifications can also be the unifications of: top and bottom (Shang Xia, 上下), left and right (Zuo You, 左右), and front and rear (Qian Hou, 前後. Six Ways means front (Qian, 前), rear (Hou, 後), left (Zuo, 左), right (You, 右), above (Shang, 上), and below (Xia, 下).

However, we must cultivate our internal spiritual understanding and then be able to manifest this understanding externally. The internal understanding includes the philosophy of Wuji, Taiji, Yin-Yang (two poles), Four Phases, Eight Trigrams, etc., how they derive or divide from one to another, and how they reunite. Moreover, we must follow the natural rules or laws so that we can reunite with nature. This is the Dao of understanding the meaning of our lives. This is also the purpose of training Taijiquan.

Chapter 4
Ten Important Keys to Taijiquan[3]

Dictated by Yang, Chen-Fu
Recorded by Chen, Wei-Ming

太極拳十要

楊澄甫口述

陳微明筆述

First, Insubstantial Jin to lead the Crown Upward.

The crown upward Jin means the appearance of the head is upright and the spirit reaches the crown. Should not allow to use force. (If) using force the crown is strong (i.e., stiff) and the Qi and blood cannot be circulating smoothly and fluidly. There must be the Yi of insubstantial, agility, and natural. Without the insubstantial Jin to lead the crown upward, then the spirit of vitality cannot be raised.

第一 · 虛領頂勁。
頂勁者，頭容正直，神貫于頂也。不可用力，用力則項
強，氣血不能流通，須有虛靈自然之意。非有虛領頂勁，
則精神不能提起也。

In a fight, the spirit (morale) must be kept high. When the spirit is high, you will be in a more alert and responsive state. The spirit also acts like a general, directing the entire battle. When a general's morale is high, his officers and soldiers will be efficiently directed. It is because of this that methods for keeping the spirit at a high level have always been an important subject in martial arts training.

In Taijiquan, the key to keeping the spirit high is first to keep the head upward, with an invisible force leading the crown upward. However, when you are doing this, you should not tense up your neck and head. If they are tensed, the blood and Qi's circulation will be stagnant. All of the suspending force should be natural and comfortable. The crucial key to reaching this goal is to pay more attention to your Yi and keep it strong, instead of using muscular force.

Second, Contain the Chest and Arc the Back.

Contain the chest means the chest contains inward slightly and allows the Qi to sink to the Dan Tian. Inhibit the chest to thrust out. (If) thrusting out, then the Qi will gather (i.e., be stagnant) at the chest area.

(Consequently,) the top is heavy and the bottom is light, the heels can easily be floating. Arcing the back means the Qi is adhering on the back (i.e., Governing Vessel). (If you) can contain the chest, then can arc the back automatically. (If you) can arc the back, then the power can be emitted from the spine. Consequently, there is no matching.

第二・含胸拔背。
含胸者，胸略內含，使氣沉于丹田也。胸忌挺出，挺出則氣擁胸際，上重下輕，腳跟易于浮起。拔背者，氣貼于背也，能含胸則自能拔背，能拔背則能力由脊發，所向無敵也。

Contain the chest and arc the back are the keys to forming Peng Jin (掤勁)(i.e., Wardoff Jin). When Peng Jin is manifested from the two arms and upper torso, defensive capability is constructed. With the Qi sunk to the Lower Dan Tian, Peng Jin will make you centered and rooted. However, your upper chest should not be tensed, even when your chest is contained and the back is arced. If this area is tensed the Qi circulation will be stagnant, the breathing will be shallow and consequently, you will be tensed and uprooted. If you can manifest Peng Jin correctly, you can store the Jin and be ready for emitting.

Third, Loosening the Waist.

The waist is the master (i.e., has control) of the entire body. (If you are) able to loosen the waist then the two feet have power and the lower disk (i.e., the root) is steady and firm. The variations of insubstantial and substantial all originate from the waist's turning and movement. Therefore, it is said: "the origin of the life (i.e., physical body) and Yi (i.e., mental body) is in the waist," "(If) there is a place without gaining the power (i.e., disadvantageous position), then find the solution from the waist and legs."

第三・鬆腰。
腰為一身之主宰，能鬆腰然后兩足有力，下盤穩固；虛
實變化皆由腰轉動，故曰：〝命意源頭在腰隙〞，〝有
不得力必于腰腿求之也。

In the book *Taiji Classic*, it is said: "The root is at the feet, (Jin or movement is) generated from the legs, mastered (i.e., controlled) by the waist and manifested (i.e., expressed) from the fingers. From the feet to the legs to the waist must be integrated, and one unified Qi." From this sentence, you can see that the waist is in control of the action. Moreover, the waist is the connection between the upper body, which manifests the Jin, and the lower body, which firms the root. Therefore, when the waist is loose, you can direct the power easily and naturally. The waist is like the steering wheel of a car. When the wheel is loose and easy to operate, you can direct the car in any direction you wish. However, if the steering wheel is stuck, then you will have difficulty moving safely and changing direction.

In addition, when the waist is loose, the connection of the upper body and the lower body will be firm. Normally, the Chinese express the root generated from the legs with the term "lower disk" (Xia Pan, 下盤). When this disk is firm, you are rooted. Furthermore, the waist area is the location of the Qi residence (i.e., Lower Dan Tian). When the waist is tensed, the Qi will not be able to enter and exit its residence easily and naturally, and you will lose the Qi support to the entire physical body's function. Therefore, when you practice Taijiquan or pushing hands, the first task is to pay attention to the waist area until you reach the stage of "regulating without regulating." That means it has become natural and comfortable.

Fourth, Discriminate Insubstantial and Substantial.

The discrimination of insubstantial and substantial is the first meaning (i.e., the most important content) in Taijiquan. If the entire body is all sitting on the right leg, then the right leg is substantial and the left leg is insubstantial. If the entire body is all sitting on the left leg, then the left leg is substantial and the right leg is insubstantial. When the insubstantial and substantial can be discriminated, then the turning and movement can be light and agile without wasting too much power. If (they) cannot be discriminated, then the stepping is heavy and stagnant, the self stance is not steady and can be pulled and moved easily by the opponent.

第四・分虛實。
太極拳術以分虛實為第一義，如全身皆坐在右腿，則右
腿為實，左腿為虛；全身皆坐在左腿，則左腿為實，右
腿為虛。虛實能分，而后轉動輕靈，毫不費力；如不能
分，則邁步重滯，自立不穩，而易為人所牽動。

Although insubstantial and substantial strategic actions can be applied everywhere in Taijiquan, this paragraph emphasizes the insubstantial and substantial only in the legs. If you can shift the weight from one leg to the other smoothly, naturally, swiftly, and comfortably, then you can maneuver your legs' insubstantial and substantial effectively. When the legs can vary as you wish, all of the insubstantial and substantial techniques based on rooting can be executed easily. However, if the leg movements are stagnant, and the exchange of insubstantial and substantial is slow, then the techniques manifested from your upper body will be slow and stagnant as well. Therefore, the capability of executing the legs' insubstantial and substantial is the key to the techniques' variations and aliveness.

Fifth, Sink the Shoulders and Drop the Elbows.

Sink the shoulders means the shoulders are loosening and hanging downward. If (you are) not able to loosen and hang down, the tip of two shoulders will be raised. Then, the Qi will follow and also raise. (In this case,) the entire body cannot gain the power. Drop the elbows means the elbows are loosening and dropping downward. (If) the elbows are suspended upward, then the shoulders will not be able to sink, (consequently,) the emitting (power) to (attack) the opponent will not be far. This is close to the broken Jin of the external family (i.e., external styles).

第五・沉肩墜肘。
沉肩者，肩鬆開下垂也。若不能鬆垂，兩肩端起，則氣亦隨之而上，全身皆不得力矣。墜肘者，肘往下鬆墜之意，肘若懸起，則肩不能沉，放人不遠，近于外家之斷勁矣。

When your shoulders and elbows are sinking and dropped, your mind moves downward. This will also lead the Qi to sink to the Lower Dan Tian and the feet to build up a firm root. In addition, when your shoulders and elbows are sunk, your arms are connected to the body with a solid foundation for the Jin's manifestation. When these two places are lifting, the Jin will be broken and not connected with the body. In this case, the Jin's manifestation would not originate from the feet, be directed by the waist, and finally be manifested from the fingers. In order to make the Jin manifest like a soft whip without interruption, the shoulders and elbows must be dropped. It is just like when you push a car; if you can drop your shoulders and elbows, your pushing force will have a root and the output will be strong. However, if you raise your shoulders and elbows, then the force manifested will be from the arms instead of the entire body, and will not be focused forward.

Sixth, Use the Yi not the Li.

The thesis of Taijiquan said: "All of these are using the Yi not the Li." (When) training Taijiquan, the entire body is loosening and opening, cannot have (even a) centimeter or millimeter's (i.e., slightly) clumsy Jin which (may cause) self bondage (i.e., clumsiness) due to the delay and stagnation (of the Qi and blood circulation) within tendons, bones, and blood. Then, (you) can be light, agile, varied, and round as wished. (You) may doubt, how can you grow power without muscular force? It is because the Jing and Luo (i.e., primary and secondary Qi channels) in the human body are like streams and ditches. When the streams and ditches are not blocked, the water will flow (smoothly), and when the Jing and Luo are not shut off, the Qi will transport (easily). If there is a stiff Jin (applied on) entire Jing and Luo (system), the Qi and blood will be stopped or stagnant and the turning and the movement will not be agile. (When this happens,) once a place is pulled, the entire body moves. If (you) do not use Li (i.e., muscular force) but use Yi, when the Yi arrives, the Qi arrives immediately. As such, then the Qi and the blood flow strongly. Transport (them) day after day until circulating the entire body without any stopping or stagnation. Practice for a long time, then (you) can gain the real internal Jin. This is what the Thesis of Taijiquan said: "Extremely soft and then (can be) extremely strong and hard." Those who have practiced Taijiquan to a proficient stage, the forearms and post-arm are like iron in cotton. Its impact is extremely heavy. Those who practice external styles, when using Li then show the Li, when not using the Li then show light and floating. Therefore, (we) can see that Li is the external Jin which is the Jin floating on the surface. If not using Yi but Li, then it is the easiest to be moved (i.e., uprooted), (therefore) it should not be encouraged.

第六・用意不用力。
太極拳論云：〝此全是用意不用力。〞練太極拳全身鬆開，不能有分毫之拙勁，以留滯于筋骨血脈之間以自縛束，然后能輕靈變化，圓轉自如。或疑不用力何以能長力？蓋人身之有經絡，如地之有溝洫，溝洫不塞而水行，經絡不閉則氣通。如渾身僵勁滿經絡，氣血停滯，轉動不靈，牽一發而全身動矣。若不用力而用意，意之所至，氣即至焉，如是氣血流注，日日貫輸，周流全身，無時停滯。久久練習，則得真正內勁，即太極拳論中所云：〝極柔軟然后極堅剛〞也。太極拳功夫純熟之人，臂膊如綿裡鐵，分量極沉；練外家拳者，用力則顯有力，不用力時，則甚輕浮，可見其力乃外勁浮面之勁也。不用意而用力，最易引動，不足尚也。

It is taught in Chinese internal martial arts that it is the Yi which leads the Qi. When this Qi is manifested physically, it is as force or power. From this, you can see that the Yi and Qi are internal, while the physical manifestation of the Yi and Qi is external. This means that the more you can concentrate, generating stronger Yi, the more abundant the generated Qi flow will be. When this abundant Qi is used to energize the physical body, the power manifestation will be stronger and more precise.

Normally, through meditation, Yi concentration can reach a higher level. Providing a relaxed body, the Qi can be circulated more smoothly and strongly. When the body is more tensed, the Qi circulation will be more stagnant. Naturally, the physical power manifested will also be dull and shallow. It is because of this that most Chinese internal martial styles emphasize the training of the meditative mind and the relaxation of the body. Often, the physical manifestation of power will not be seen until after the Qi has been led from the Lower Dan Tian sufficiently. However, in most of the external styles, the meditative mind receives little attention. Moreover the relaxation of the physical body to provide smooth Qi circulation is commonly ignored. Often, the physical body is tensed too early and the Qi's circulation becomes stagnant. It is because of this that almost all internal martial styles focus on the training of Yi instead of Li.

Seventh, the Top and the Bottom Mutually Follow Each Other.

The top and the bottom mutually following each other is what the Thesis of Taijiquan said: "Its root is in the feet, originated from the legs, mastered at the waist, and manifested in the fingers. From the feet to the legs and to the waist, all must be integrated with a sole Qi." The hands move, the waist moves, the feet move, the eyes' spirit (i.e., sense of enemy) also follow to move. As such, then it can be said the top and the bottom mutually follow each other. (If) there is a place without moving, then it is disordered.

第七・上下相隨。
上下相隨者，即太極拳論中所云：〝其跟在腳，發于腿，
主宰于腰，形于手指，由腳而腿而腰，總須完整一氣〞
也。手動、腰動、足動，眼神亦隨之動，如是方可謂之
上下相隨，有一不動，即散亂也。

This paragraph talks about the integration of the mind (i.e., spirit) and body. When the mind and the body can be integrated as a single fighting unit, every part of the body will coordinate and harmonize with all others. All of this depends on the continuous circulation of the Qi, which threads from the feet to the fingers. Moreover, in order to make the Qi circulate smoothly and fluidly, the entire body must act as a soft whip. The Jin manifested in Taijiquan is like Jin manifested by a soft whip. In order to make the whipping power strong, all of the joints must be relaxed and loose, and the movement and energy must thread into a single whipping instant. If there is any tiny place in the joints that is tensed and tightened, then the whipping force will be hindered.

Success in this depends on the feeling. Feeling is the language of the mind and the body. When your sensitivity is deep and profound, you can bring your softness and relaxation to the deepest place. This means you can be softer than other people, and the Qi can circulate more smoothly and fluidly than others. Because of this, all of the internal martial styles emphasize training the deeply concentrated mind (i.e., meditative mind), which enables you to reach a deeper sensitivity of feeling. The stronger your concentration, the higher your spirit will be.

Eighth, Internal and External Harmonize (Unify) with Each Other.

What Taijiquan trains is the spirit. Therefore it is said: "The spirit is the commanding general and the body is the emissary." (If) the spirit of vitality can be raised, automatically the movements will be light and agile. The postures are nothing else but insubstantial, substantial, opening, and closing. What the opening means is that not only the hands and feet can open, the Xin (i.e., emotional mind) and Yi (i.e., wisdom mind) can also be open at the same time. What the closing means it that not only the hands and feet can close, the Xin and Yi can also close at the same time. (If) the internal and external can be unified as a sole Qi, then (the Taijiquan will be) complete without any gap.

第八・內外相合。
太極拳所練在神，故云：〝神為主帥，身為驅使〞。精神能提得起，自然舉動輕靈。架子不外虛實開合。所謂開者，不但手足開，心意亦與之俱開。所謂合者，不但手足合，心意亦與之俱合。能內外合為一氣，則渾然無間矣。

In internal martial arts, not only are integrity of the mind and external physical manifestation seriously emphasized, but so is the unification and harmony of the internal and external. Internal means the mind (i.e., the spirit) and the Qi, and external means the physical structure and strength. You should always remember that it is the Yi (i.e., mind) which leads the Qi to the physical body for manifestation. If this process can be executed harmoniously, then the manifestation of the internal Yi and Qi into the external physical form can be efficient and effective. When the mind is strong, the spirit can be raised to a proficient level. Alertness and awareness will be enhanced and the morale will also be lifted to a higher level. When this happens, your physical body can execute the mind's decisions precisely and responsively. The entire body's internal and external can then perform as an efficient fighting unit.

Ninth, Continuous without Broken.

In the external fists techniques (i.e., external martial skills), the Jins manifested are the Post-Heaven's (i.e., after birth) clumsy Jins. Therefore, there is a beginning and an end. (When) there is continuity and breakage, the old Li (i.e., muscular force) has already ended and the new Li has not yet been generated. This is the moment that can be attacked easiest. Taijiquan uses the Yi without using the Li. From the beginning until the end, continuous without breaking, (when) complete, again repeated from beginning, cycling without limitation. It is what was originally said: "Like the long great river (i.e., Yangtze river), flow fluidly without ending." It is also said: "Transporting the Jin as drawing the silk." All of this means the (movements) are threaded through (i.e., together) with a sole Qi.

第九・相連不斷。
外家拳術，其勁乃后天之拙勁，故有起有止，有續有斷，
舊力已盡，新力未生，此時最易為人所乘。太極拳用意
不用力，自始至終，綿綿不斷，周而復始，循環無窮。
原所謂「如長江大河，滔滔不絕，」又曰「運勁如抽
絲」，皆言其貫串一氣也。

One of the special characteristics of Taijiquan is its continuity of the mind, Qi circulation, and action. The ending movement of the previous action is the beginning movement of the next action. From the skills of Listening Jin (Ting Jin, 聽勁), Following Jin (Sui Jin, 隨勁), Attaching Jin (Zhan Jin, 粘勁), Adhering Jin (Nian Jin, 黏勁, and Connecting Jin (Lian Jin, 連勁), you can control the entire action and respond to the opponent's action with continuity. In fact, this is one of the most special and important trainings in Chinese soft martial styles. This is very different from the training of the external martial arts, which focus on the execution of individual techniques, that can result in no connection between techniques. Taijiquan can therefore use the strategy of defense as an offense effectively and efficiently.

Tenth, Seeking for Calmness in the Movements.

The fist techniques (i.e., martial skills) of the external styles grant expertise in jumping and walking, use the

Qi and Li until it is exhausted. Therefore, right after practice, nobody without panting. Taijiquan uses the calmness to control the movements, though moving remain calm. Therefore, when practicing postures, (it is) the slower the better. When slow, then the breathing is deep and long, the Qi is sunk to Dan Tian. Consequently, there is no harmful problem like the blood vessels' expansion. The practitioners should ponder and comprehend it carefully, then can (they) obtain its meaning.

第十・動中求靜。

外家拳術，以跳躍為能，用盡氣力，故練習之后，無不喘氣者。太極拳以靜御動，雖動尤靜，故練架子愈慢愈好。慢則呼吸深長，氣沉丹田，自無血脈償張之弊。學者細心休會，庶可得其意焉。

One of the main differences between Taijiquan and other external martial styles is that Taijiquan uses defense as offense, and uses calmness to handle movement. The spending of energy is conserved, and therefore fighting endurance can be extensive. In addition, when you are calm, your physical body will be relaxed, and consequently oxygen consumption is minimized. However, the most important element of all is that Taijiquan emphasizes long, profound breathing techniques that allow you to take in plenty of oxygen for action. It is because of this that it is not like external styles, which can leave you short of breath after fighting for only a short time.

From a health conscious perspective, when you are relaxed and calm, the physical body will be serene. This will provide the best condition for the blood and Qi circulation. In this manner, hypertension can be eased, the heart-beat slowed down, and high blood pressure can be lowered. All of these benefits can only be comprehended and experienced by those Taijiquan practitioners who have practiced for some time. As long as you keep pondering and practicing, sooner or later, you will gain these experiences.

Chapter 5
Explanation of Taijiquan's Harmonious Stepping in Four Sides of Pushing Hands[3]

Yang, Chen-Fu

太極拳合步四正推手解 楊澄甫

Taijiquan uses pushing hands practice as the applications. Learning pushing hands means learning Feeling Jin. When there is Feeling Jin, then Understanding Jin is not difficult. Therefore, The Total Thesis (of Taijiquan) said: "from Understanding Jin then gradually reach the spiritual enlightenment." There is no doubt that this sentence is rooted in (built upon) pushing hands. Peng (i.e., Wardoff), Lu (i.e., Rollback), Ji (i.e., Press), and An (i.e., Push), four (Jin) patterns are the stationary pushing hands of adhering, connecting, attaching, and following which give up self and follow the opponent.

太極拳以練習推手為致用，學推手則即是學覺勁，有覺勁則懂勁便不難矣。故總論所謂由懂勁而階及神明，此言即根於推手無疑矣。掤、攦、擠、按四式即黏、連、貼、隨舍己從人之定步推手。

After you have completed Taijiquan practice and understand the dynamics of the postures, then you can advance forward into the applications. The main training method for understanding and mastering Taijiquan applications is through pushing hands practice. Practically speaking, in order to make all of the Taijiquan techniques effective and useful, you must first comprehend and master the skills of adhering (Nian, 黏), connecting (Lian, 連), attaching (Tie or Zhan, 貼·粘), and following (Sui, 隨). However, the success of executing all of these techniques depends on how sensitively you can feel into yourself and your opponent. This sensitive feeling is called "Listening Jin" (Ting Jin, 聽勁) which means the listening of the skin through touch, or even without touching. Once you have achieved a profound level of "Listening Jin," then are you able to understand the opponent's intention (i.e., "Understanding Jin," Dong Jin, 懂勁). Only through this communication can you then execute your techniques skillfully. The more you practice, the higher the level of sensitivity you will obtain. After you have reached a proficient level, then even before your opponent's action is initiated, you will already sense his intention and be ready for it. This stage means you have reached enlightenment in pushing hands.

The technique of Peng is outward. It is used to defend against the opponent's An so (he) is not able to apply (his) An to close (my) chest and abdomen. Therefore it is called "Peng" (i.e., Wardoff). To adopt the meaning of this Peng word, it is slightly different from the expatiation in the article's explanation. The methods of Peng, the left and right use the same methods and most taboo in stiffness and stagnation. (Ambiguity in original document) When stiff, (I) do not know the movements of myself. When stagnant, (then, I) do not know the opponent's attacking and retreating. If (I) do not know myself and also do not know the opponent, then it is not pushing hands. If there is delay and heaviness, then it means Li (i.e., muscular force) has been used to defend against the opponent. This has become dead hands (i.e., clumsy techniques) and are not desired by the Taiji family (i.e., style). Peng must be adhering instead of resisting. (Though) the arms are Peng outward, the Yi wishes to adhere and retreat and again not wish to allow (my) Peng hands too close to (my) chest. (Therefore, I) must use Neutralizing Jin by relying on the waist's turning. Once the waist is turned, then my Peng's formation has been completed.

掤法向外，駕禦敵人之按手，使不得按至胸腹貼近。故曰掤。此掤字取意，與說文釋義稍異。掤之方式，左右同其用法，最忌板滯。板者，不知自己之運動。滯者，不知敵人之取舍。既不知己，又不知彼，則不成為推手矣。遲重者，必以力禦人，便成死手，非太極家之所取也。必曰掤者，黏也非抗也。手向外掤，意欲黏回，又不使己之掤手與胸部貼近。得化勁全賴轉腰，一轉腰則我之掤勢已成矣。

Taijiquan is also called "Thirteen Postures" (Shi San Shi, 十三勢). Though it has been translated as "Thirteen Postures," in fact, it covers the eight most basic Taijiquan Jin patterns, which are called "Eight Doors" (Ba Men, 八門), and the five kinds of strategic stepping which are called "Five Steppings" (Wu Bu, 五步). Among these thirteen Jin patterns and five strategic steppings, Peng Jin (掤勁) is the first and the most basic but most important Jin pattern. Peng Jin can be found in almost all of the Taijiquan postures. This is because Peng Jin allows you to construct a defensive posture and yet provides you with a good opportunity and posture for Jin manifestation.

The word Peng, in fact, cannot be found in a typical Chinese dictionary. It was created in Chinese martial arts. This word is constructed from the characters for hand (扌) and for two moons (月). The moon around the earth is single and therefore lonely. When two moons are together, then there is a companion and it means friends (朋) in Chinese. Since there is friendship, it means to harmonize, to coordinate, and to cooperate with each other. Therefore, Peng means using the arms to form two moons that coordinate with each other. However, the Jin pattern of Peng must also include the roundness of the chest. Its passing oral secret is "containing the chest and arc the back" (Han Xiong Ba Bei, 含胸拔背). That means a round expansive Jin is constructed from the two arms and the upper chest.

When this Jin is constructed, you will firm your center, which protects you from your opponent's pressing and pushing against your chest and abdomen. Moreover, from the formation of this Jin pattern, you have stored the Jin in the posture for further emitting.

Though Peng Jin is powerful and can help you defend yourself effectively, however, it is very easy for a beginner to be tensed and become stiff. Once you commit this mistake, your technique will be clumsy and the feeling (i.e., Listening Jin) will be stagnant. Therefore, the key to performing correct Peng Jin is to be hard (i.e., strong) externally but soft internally. To reach this goal, you must know the trick of "Yielding Jin" (Rang Jin, 讓勁) and also the maneuver of "Turning Jin (Zhuan Jin, 轉勁). Once you have these two key skills, you can be soft yet strong.

Lu, means to connect (through) the opponent's elbow and wrist, without resisting and without plucking. This is because when the opponent extends his arm to attack me, I follow his coming posture and take him. This is the mind of taking it back (i.e., lead it backward) and is called Lu (i.e., Rollback). This word is again different from the elucidation of the article. It is a special terminology used in the fist techniques family (i.e., martial art society). Its method is a rollback with the waist's turning in addition to the connection of one hand with the opponent's elbow. The person being rollback (rolled back) must comply with (the theory) of giving up himself and following the opponent. (He) must also know where (he) is able to give up the opponent and follow himself. (For example,) when (I am being) rollback and feel the pressure is getting heavy, then (I) may take the opportunity and use (my) Kao (i.e., Bump). However, (if I) feel the opponent's Rollback Jin is suddenly continuous and broken, then immediately give up (i.e., ignore) his one side and attack with a press.

攦者，連著彼之肘與腕，不抗不採。因彼伸臂襲我，我
順其勢而取之。是收回意謂之攦。此字義又與說文不同，
乃拳術家之專用名詞也。其方法即攦法轉腰加上一手連
著彼之肘節間。被攦者須本舍己從人，亦須知有舍人從
己之處。被攦覺其手加重，便可乘之以靠。或覺其攦勁，
忽有斷續，則急舍其一邊，而襲以擠可也。

When you apply the Jin pattern of rollback (Lu, 攦), one of your hands is connecting with the opponent's wrist while the other is connecting with his elbow. In this case, whenever it is proper or necessary, you may immediately apply Pluck Jin (Cai, 採勁) to control these two places. However, if there is no special intention for plucking, then you simply follow the opponent's incoming force and lead it to the side. Lu Jin includes Yielding Jin (Rang Jin, 讓勁), Leading Jin (Yin Jin, 引勁), and Neutralizing Jin (Hua Jin, 化勁. The oral secret of applying Lu Jin is "to lead the Jin into emptiness" (Yin Jin Luo Kong, 引勁落空). Again, this word would not be found in a traditional Chinese dictionary. It was created by Chinese martial arts. When you apply Lu Jin, first you must yield (i.e., listen and follow). This will trick your opponent's mind to continue his action. Then you use your waist's turning to lead the incoming force to the side and finally take it into emptiness. From this, you can see that the turning of the waist is the key to successful execution of Lu Jin. The waist is the control center that directs the power generated from the legs in the desired direction.

However, if your opponent is applying Lu Jin to you, you should not resist. Once you resist, your tensed body will connect your arm back to your root. When this happens, your opponent can change his strategy and use Press Jin (Ji Jin, 擠勁) or Bump Jin (Kao Jin, 靠勁) to make you lose your balance easily. The way of handling the situation of being rolled back is, when you feel the opponent's rollback press has increased, simply follow this action, twist your elbow slightly and bend to escape from the elbow lock, immediately follow with Press Jin or Kao Jin. However, if you feel your opponent's Rollback Jin is not continuous, you have an opportunity to catch the proper timing to press or bump him.

Ji, is just opposite from Lu. Lu is to induce the opponent's An Jin and make him enter my trap to be taken. This will be victory for sure. (However,) assume that my moving force is felt (i.e., detected) first by the opponent, then his advancing Jin (i.e., An Jin) will be broken and changed into another posture (i.e., action). In this case, the action of my Lu will be ineffective and therefore, (I) cannot but change my retreating into advancing. Use (my) front hand to pluck his elbow from sideways, move (my) rear hand and add it to the forearm of the front hand and take the opportunity to press forward. Then, there is no opponent, when encountering this sudden change, will not lose his advantageous situation and (be) pressed out by me. If the person being pressed is able to (be) calm and steady in this sudden change, (also) has a prior feeling and immediately empties the coming Ji Jin, then (he) can change the situation into An Jin (i.e., push down or press down).

擠者，正與攦式相反。攦則誘彼敵之按勁，使其進而入
我陷阱而取之，必勝矣。設我之動力，先為彼所覺，則
彼進勁必中斷，而變為他式，則我之攦勢失效，則不可
不反退為進。用前手側採其肘，提起後手，加在前手小
臂內便乘勢擠出。則彼倉猝變化之中，未有不失其機勢，
而被我擠出矣。被擠者須於變化中能鎮定，有先覺，急
空其擠勁，則便成其按勢矣。

Ji (擠) means to press or to squeeze. When Ji Jin is applied in pushing hands, often press action is adopted. Ji Jin and Lu Jin (攦勁) (i.e., Rollback Jin) are commonly used together and are exchangeable from one to the other. Ji is to advance, more aggressive and more Yang, while Lu is to neutralize, is more defensive and more Yin. For example, when you use Lu Jin on the opponent's arm, if the opponent has noticed your intention, he will immediately stop his advancing force to avoid his force being led into emptiness. That means his Jin is broken. When this happens, it will provide you with a great opportunity to change your Lu Jin into Ji Jin and press him off balance. In order to execute your Ji Jin successfully, your hand on his elbow will change into Cai Jin (採勁)(i.e., Pluck Jin) to immobilize his elbow from further action while placing your other hand on the inner forearm of the plucking arm to press him/off balance. The key to performing this strategy depends on correct timing.

However, if you are in the position of being Ji (i.e., pressed), in order to escape your awkward situation, you must remain calm and be ready for the sudden change. In order to neutralize the Ji Jin your opponent is applying, you must also use An Jin (按勁)(i.e., Press Down) to press his arm down. In this case, the incoming pressing force will be neutralized.

An, because the Ji cannot gain its advantageous situation, then place (your) right hand in attaching on the opponent's left external elbow on the turning area, then change into Lu posture and rollback. If Rollback cannot gain advantageous situation, then turn the right hand and use the center of the palm to push downward on the opponent's elbow joint. Again, the left hand uses

the center of the left palm to push down on the oppo-
nent's left wrist. This is called An (i.e., Push or
Downward). After An, again change into Peng. Peng,
Lu, Ji, and An complete and again repeat, cycle with-
out ceasing. This is the meaning of practicing adhering,
connecting, attaching, and following. The variations of
the above four patterns are unlimited. It is hard to
describe by the pen. Hope the practitioner comprehend
them carefully.

按者，因擠式不得其機勢，便將右手，緣彼敵之左肘外
廉轉上，仍成攦式履回。如攦又不得勢，則翻右手，以
手心按彼左肘節上抽出。左手又以手心按彼左腕上，是
謂之按。按之轉復為掤。掤攦擠按終而復始，輪轉不息。
此謂練習黏連貼隨之意也。以上四式，變化無窮，筆難
縷術，望學者幸細心領會。

An Jin (按勁)(i.e., Press or Push Downward Jin) is commonly
used against the opponent's Ji (擠)(i.e., Press) and Kao (靠)(i.e.,
Bump). When An is used against these two Jin patterns, the joints
such as the shoulders, elbows, and/or wrists are normally the places
to be pushed down to seal the opponent's arm's further action.

In a real situation, if you fail to execute your Ji successfully—for
example, when the opponent has used his Peng to build up his center and firm his root, then it will be difficult for you to apply Ji. In this
case, you should immediately change into Lu to destroy his/her center and balance. Then, you apply An right away to seal his arm down
for your further attack. Alternatively, you may immediately use An to
your opponent's chest to push him off balance.

From this discussion, you can see that Peng, Lu, Ji, and An are
mutually subduing and supportive of each other. Therefore, they can
be practiced continuously. In Taijiquan pushing hands practice, it is
commonly called "double pushing hands" (Shuang Tui Shou,
雙推手). As long as you keep practicing these four basic Jin patterns,
you will soon become proficient in your adhering, connecting,
attaching, and following skills.

References

1. 太極拳・刀、劍、桿、散手合編，陳炎林著。

2. 太極拳術，顧留馨著，上海體育出版社, 1992.

3. 楊澄甫式太極拳，楊振基口述，嚴翰秀整理，廣西民族出, 1993.

4. 楊禹廷太極拳系列、秘要集錦，李秉慈、翁福麒編著，奧林匹克
   出版社, 1990.

5. 太極拳全書，人民體育出版社, 1988.

6. 太極拳講義，吳公藻編，上海書店, 1985.

7. *Lost T'ai-chi Classics from the Late Ch'ing Dynasty*, Douglas Wile, 1996.

8. 陰陽不必分男女，體氣強弱即陰陽。

9. 兩個男人可栽接，一對女人能採補。

Translation and Glossary of Chinese Terms

An 按 Means "pressing or stamping." One of the eight basic moving or Jin patterns of Taijiquan. These eight moving patterns are called "Ba Men" (八門) which means "eight doors." When An is done, first relax the wrist and when the hand has reached the opponent's body, immediately settle down the wrist. This action is called "Zuo Wan" (坐腕) in Taijiquan practice.

An Jin 按勁 The martial power generated from the An moving pattern of Taijiquan.

Ba Gua (Ba Kua) 八卦 Literally, "Eight Divinations." Also called the Eight Trigrams. In Chinese philosophy, the eight basic variations; shown in the *Yi Jing* (易經)(*Book of Change*) as groups of single and broken lines.

Ba Kua Chang (Baguazhang) 八卦掌 Means "Eight Trigram Palms." The name of one of the Chinese internal martial styles.

Ba Men 八門 Means "eight doors." The art of Taijiquan is constructed from eight basic moving or Jin patterns and the five basic steppings. The eight basic moving or Jin patterns that can be used to handle the eight directions of action are called the "eight doors" and the five stepping actions are called the "five steppings."

Ba Men Wu Bu 八門五步 Means "eight doors and five steppings." The art of Taijiquan is constructed from eight basic moving or Jin patterns and the five basic steppings. The eight basic moving or Jin patterns that can be used to handle the eight directions of action are called the "eight doors," and the five stepping actions are called the "five steppings."

Bagua 八卦 Literally, "Eight Divinations." Also called the Eight Trigrams. In Chinese philosophy, the eight basic variations; shown in the *Yi Jing* as groups of single and broken lines.

Baguazhang (Ba Kua Zhang) 八卦掌 Means "Eight Trigram Palms." The name of one of the Chinese internal martial styles.

Bai He 白鶴 White Crane. A style of Chinese martial arts.

Bi 閉 Means "close" or "seal."

Bi Xue 閉穴 To seal the cavities. One of the highest levels of skills in Chinese martial arts.

Bian 匾 Deficiency.

Biao Li 表裡 Means "surface and internal." Surface means skin while internal means internal organs.

Cai 採 Plucking.

Cai Jin 採勁 The martial power of plucking.

Can Si Jin Chan Shou Lian Xi 纏絲勁纏手練習 Silk reeling Jin coiling training. One of the important basic trainings in Taijiquan.

Chan 纏 To wrap or to coil. A common Chinese martial arts technique.

Chan Jin 纏勁 The martial power of wrapping or coiling.

Chang Chuan (Changquan) 長拳 Means "long range fist or long sequence." Chang Chuan includes all northern Chinese long range martial styles. Taijiquan is also called Chang Chuan simply because its sequence is long.

Chang Jiang 長江 Literally, long river. Refers to the Yangtze river (揚子江) in southern China.

Chang Ju 長距 Means "long range or long distance."

Changquan (Chang Chuan) 長拳 Means "long range fist or long sequence." Chang Chuan includes all northern Chinese long range martial styles. Taijiquan is also called Chang Chuan simply because its sequence is long.

Chen Jia Gou 陳家溝 Chen's village, where Chen style Taijiquan originated.

Chen, Chang-Xing 陳長興 Yang, Lu-Shan's master. A well known Chen style Taijiquan master during the Qi dynasty.

Chen, Yan-Lin 陳炎林 A well known Taijiquan master in China during the 1940's who wrote a book entitled, *Tai Chi Chuan: Saber, Sword, Staff, and Sparring*, (太極拳，刀、劍、桿、散手合編), Reprinted in Taipei, Taiwan, 1943.

Cheng, Gin-Gsao 曾金灶 Dr. Yang, Jwing-Ming's White Crane master.

Cheng, Man-Ching 鄭曼清 A well known Chinese Taijiquan master in America during the 1960's.

Chengjiang (Co-24) 承漿 An acupuncture cavity located on the face.

Chi (Qi) 氣 The energy pervading the universe, including the energy circulating in the human body.

Chi Kung (Qigong) 氣功 The Gongfu of Qi, which means the study of Qi.

Chin Na (Qin Na) 擒拿 Literally means "seize control." A component of Chinese martial arts which emphasizes grabbing techniques, to control your opponent's joints, in conjunction with attacking certain acupuncture cavities.

Confucius 孔子 A Chinese scholar, during the period of 551-479 B.C., whose philosophy has significantly influenced Chinese culture.

Cui 捶 Pounding.

Cuo 挫、搓 Filing.

Da 打 Striking. Normally, to attack with the palms, fists or arms.

Da Quan 大圈 Large circle. One of the common fighting distances.

Dan Tian 丹田 "Elixir field." Located in the lower abdomen. It is considered the place which can store Qi energy.

Dao 道 The "way," by implication the "natural way."

Dao De Jing 道德經 *Morality Classic.* Written by Lao Zi (老子) during the Zhou Dynasty (1122-934 B.C.)(周朝).

Dao Jia 道家 The Dao family. Daoism. Created by Lao Zi during the Zhou Dynasty (1122-934 B.C.). In the Han Dynasty (c. 58 A.D.)(漢朝), it was mixed with Buddhism to become the Daoist religion (Dao Jiao)(道教).

Dian 點 "To point" or "to press."

Dian Mai (Dim Mak) 點脈 Mai means "the blood vessel" (Xue Mai)(穴脈) or "the Qi channel" (Qi Mai)(氣脈). Dian Mai means "to press the blood vessel or Qi channel."

Dian Xue 點穴 Dian means "to point and exert pressure" and Xue means "the cavities." Dian Xue refers to those Qin Na techniques which specialize in attacking acupuncture cavities to immobilize or kill an opponent.

Dihe (M-HN-19) 地合 An acupuncture cavity located on the face.

Ding 頂 Butting.

Diu 丢 Losing.

Dong 動 Moving.

Dong Jin 懂勁 "Understanding Jin." One of the Jins which uses the feeling of the skin to sense the opponent's energy.

Duan 斷 "To break" or "to seal."

Duan Ju 短距 Means "short range." A common fighting distance in which you and your opponent can reach each other with your hands.

Duan Mai 斷脈 Duan means "to break" and Mai means "the blood vessel." Duan Mai means "to seal or to break the blood vessel."

Dui 兌 One of the Eight Trigrams.

Fa Chuan 化拳 Literally, neutralizing fist, or neutralizing style. It is called this because its motions are soft and able to neutralize the opponent's power.

Fu 俯 To lean or bend forward.

Fu Xi (2852-2737 B.C.) 伏羲 The first important and unifying ancestor of the Chinese Han race (漢族).

Gen 艮 One of the Eight Trigrams.

Gong (Kung) 功 Energy or hard work.

Gongfu (Kung Fu) 功夫 Means "energy-time." Anything which will take time and energy to learn or to accomplish is called Gongfu.

Gu 顧 To look around, to be aware of, or to pay attention.

Gu Jing 固精 To firm the essence.

Gung Li Chuan 功力拳 The name of a barehand sequence in Chinese Long Fist martial arts.

Guoshu 國術 Abbreviation of "Zhongguo Wushu" (中國武術) which means "Chinese Martial Techniques."

Ha 哈 A Yang sound that is used to manifest martial power to its highest efficiency.

Han 漢 A dynasty in Chinese history (206 B.C.-221 A.D.)

Han race 漢族 The major race in China.

Han Xiong Ba Bei 含胸拔背 Means to contain or draw in the chest and arc the back.

Han, Ching-Tang 韓慶堂 A well known Chinese martial artist, especially in Taiwan in the last forty years. Master Han is also Dr. Yang Jwing-Ming's Long Fist grandmaster.

He 合 Means "to close."

Hen 哼 A Yin Qigong sound that is the opposite of the Yang Ha sound. This sound is commonly used to lead the Qi inward and to store it in the bone marrow. This sound can also be used for an attack when the manifestation of only partial power is desired.

Heng Shan 衡山 Heng mountain. One of the five sacred mountains in China located in Heng Shan County, Hunan province (湖南省·衡山縣). It is also called "Nan Yue" (南嶽) and means "south mountain."

Heng Shan 恆山 Heng mountain. One of the five sacred mountains in China located in Hebei and Shanxi provinces (河北省，山西省). It is also called "Bei Yue" (北嶽) and means "north mountain."

Hou 後 Rear.

Hua 化 "To neutralize."

Hua Jin 化勁 The Jin (martial power) used to neutralize the opponent's attacking.

Hua Shan 華山 Hua mountain. One of the five sacred mountains in China located in Hua Yin county, Shanxi province (陝西省·華陰縣). It is also called "Xi Yue" (西嶽) and means "west mountain."

Huai He 淮河 Huai river. One of the four great rivers in China.

Huan 換 To exchange or to alter.

Huan 緩 To slow down.

Huan 還 To return (i.e., to turn back).

Huang He 黃河 Yellow River. One of the four great rivers in China.

Hubei province 湖北省 One of the provinces in southern China.

Huo 火 Fire. One of the five elements in the Five Phases.

Ji 急 Means urgent, rapid, or fast.

Ji 擠 Means "to squeeze" or "to press."

Ji He 濟河 Ji river. One of the four great rivers in China.

Ji Jin 擠勁 The martial power of pressing or squeezing.

Jiang 降 To fall, to drop, or to descend.

Jie 接 Means "to connect."

Jie 結 Knots or congealment (i.e., stagnation).

Jie Mo 節膜 To control or to check the fasciae. Filing is a crucial skill that can be used to damage the opponent's fasciae.

Jin 金 Metal. One of the five elements in the Five Phases.

Jin 進 Advance or step forward.

Jin (Jing) 勁 Chinese martial power. A combination of "Li" (muscular power) and "Qi."

Jin Bu 進步 Means "to step forward."

Jin, Shao-Feng 金紹峰   Master Yang Jwing-Ming's White Crane grandmaster.

Jin-Li 勁力 Means martial power.

Jing 靜 Calm.

Jing 精 Essence. The most refined part of anything.

Jing (Jin) 勁 Chinese martial power. A combination of "Li" (力)(muscular power) and "Qi" (氣).

Kai 開 To open.

Kan 坎 One of the Eight Trigrams, meaning "water." Referred to in "Kan and Li (fire)."

Kang 抗 To resist.

Kao 靠 Means "to lean or to press against." In Taijiquan, it means to bump someone off balance.

Kao Jin 靠勁 The martial power of bumping.

Kao, Tao 高濤 Dr. Yang, Jwing-Ming's first Taijiquan master.

Kong 空 Empty or void.

Kong Men 空門 Empty doors. The doors you can step in to initiate an effective attack.

Kun 坤 One of the Eight Trigrams.

Kung (Gong) 功 Means "energy" or "hard work."

Kung Fu (Gongfu) 功夫 Means "energy-time." Anything which will take time and energy to learn or to accomplish is called Kung Fu.

Li 力 The power which is generated from muscular strength.

Li 理 Natural rules and principles.

Li 離 One of the Eight Trigrams, meaning "fire." Referred to in "Kan (water) and Li."

Li, Mao-Ching 李茂清 Dr. Yang, Jwing-Ming's Long Fist master.

Lian 連 To connect.

Lian Jin 連勁 The martial power of connecting.

Liao 撩 Provoking (i.e., inciting).

Lie 挒 Means "to rend" or "to split."

Lie Jin 挒勁 The martial power of "rend."

Lien Bu Chuan 連步拳 One of the Long Fist barehand sequences.

Lin, Bo-Yuan 林伯原 An author who wrote the book, *Chinese Wushu History* (中國武術史), Wu Zhou Publications (五洲出版社), Taipei, 1996.

Lu 攦 Means "to rollback."

Lu Jin 攦勁 The martial power of rolling backward (rollback).

Luo 落 To descend, to fall, or to lower.

Ma Bu 馬步 Horse stance. One of the basic stances trained in Chinese martial arts.

Mai 脈 Means "vessel" or "Qi channel."

Mao 卯 One of the twelve Terrestrial Branches (i.e., 5-7 A.M.).

Mi 米 Rice.

Mian Quan 綿拳 Literally, cotton fist. It means soft style. Taijiquan is also called Mian Quan.

Miao Hou 眇後 Peeking to the rear.

Mingmen 命門 Literally, life doors. In this book, it means the two kidneys.

Mo 摩 Scouring is a quick frictional movement on the opponent's skin. This action allows you to move from one place to another without losing contact with the opponent.

Mu 木 Wood. One of the Five Elements.

Na 拿 Means "to hold" or "to grab." However, when Na is applied in Taijiquan, it is a technique in which you use your hands to stick with the opponent's joints so as to immobilize his further action.

Na Mai 拿脈 Seizing the Qi or blood vessels.

Nanking Central Guoshu Institute 南京中央國術館 A national martial arts institute organized by the Chinese government in 1928.

Nei Wai 內外 Means internal thinking and external action (i.e., mind and body).

Nian 黏 To stick or to adhere.

Nian Jin 黏勁 The martial power of adhering.

Pan 盼 To look or to be aware of.

Peng 掤 Means "to ward off."

Peng Jin 掤勁 The martial power of warding off.

Qi 起   To ascend or to rise.

Qi (Chi) 氣   Chinese term for universal energy. A current popular model is that the Qi circulating in the human body is bioelectric in nature.

Qian 乾   One of the Eight Trigrams.

Qian 前   Front.

Qian Hou 前後   Means "front and rear."

Qigong (Chi Kung) 氣功   The Gongfu of Qi, which means the study of Qi.

Qimen (Li-14) 期門   An acupuncture cavity belonging to the Liver Channel.

Qin (Chin) 擒   Means "to catch" or "to seize."

Qin Na (Chin Na) 擒拿   Literally means "seize control." A component of Chinese martial arts which emphasizes grabbing techniques to control your opponent's joints, in conjunction with attacking certain acupuncture cavities.

Qiu 酉   One of the twelve Terrestrial Branches (i.e., 5-7 P.M.).

Qu 屈   To bend.

Quan 圈   Circle.

Rang Jin 讓勁   Yielding Jin. The martial power that is used to yield to incoming force.

Renzhong (Gv-26) 人中   An acupuncture cavity under the nose.

Rou 柔、揉   Circle rubbing is a circular rubbing action using the palm or the base of the palm to press the opponent and then rub in with circles. Circle rubbing is commonly used for massage. It can also be used to damage the opponent's fasciae when the power and the techniques are applied accurately. It can also be used to attack the cavities when the knuckle of a finger is used.

San Bao 三寶   Three treasures. Essence (Jing)(精), energy (Qi)(氣) and spirit (Shen)(神). Also called San Yuan (three origins).

San Cai 三才   Three powers. Heaven, Earth and Man.

San Jiao 三教   Means three schools. The three schools are Buddhism, Daoism, and Confucianism.

Shan 閃   Means "to dodge."

Shang 上   Means "above," "top," or "upper."

Shang Xia 上下 Top and bottom.

Shen 神 Spirit. According to Chinese Qigong, the Shen resides at the Upper Dan Tian (the third eye).

Shen 伸 Means "to extend."

Sheng 升 Means "to raise."

Shi Er Di Zhi 十二地支 The Twelve Terrestrial Branches or Horary Characters which include: Zi (子)(11 P.M.-1 A.M.)-Rat, Chou (丑)(1-3 A.M.)-Ox, Yin (寅)(3-5 A.M.)-Tiger, Mao (卯)(5-7 A.M.)-Hare, Chen (辰)(7-9 A.M.)-Dragon, Yi (巳)(9-11A.M.)-Snake, Wu (午)(11A.M.-1 P.M.)-Horse, Wei (未)(1-3 P.M.)-Sheep, Shen (申)(3-5 P.M.)-Monkey, Qiu (酉)(5-7 P.M.)-Cock, Shu (戌)(7-9 P.M.)-Dog, and Hai (亥)(9-11 P.M.)-Boar.

Shi San Shi 十三勢 Means "Thirteen Postures." Taijiquan is also called "Thirteen Postures." It is simply because Taijiquan is built upon eight Jin patterns and five strategic movements.

Shi Tian Gan 十天干 The Ten Celestial Stems, which include: Jia (甲), Yi (乙), Bing (丙), Ding (丁), Wu (戊), Ji (己), Geng (庚), Xin (辛), Ren (壬), and Gui (癸).

Shou Jiao 手腳 Hands and feet.

Shuang Tui Shou 雙推手 Double pushing hands. A two person's matching training in Taijiquan for Peng (掤), Lu (攦), Ji (擠), and An (按).

Shuang Zhong 雙重 Means "double weighting or double layering." It means when the opponent has placed a weight or pressure on you, and you respond by meeting that pressure with equal or greater pressure of your own. The consequence is stagnation. When this happens, mutual resistance will be generated.

Shui 水 Water. One of the Five Elements.

Song Shan 嵩山 Song mountain. One of the five sacred mountains in China, located in Deng Feng county, Henan province (河南省·登封縣). It is also called "Zhong Yue" (中嶽) and means "central mountain."

Sui 隨 Means "to follow."

Sui Jin 隨勁 Following Jin. The martial power which is used to follow the opponent's action.

Tai Chi Chuan (Taijiquan) 太極拳 A Chinese internal martial style which is based on the theory of Taiji (grand ultimate).

Tai Shan 泰山   Tai mountain. One of the five sacred mountains in China, located in Tai An county, Shandong province (山東省・泰安縣).

Taiji 太極   Means "grand ultimate." It is this force which generates two poles, Yin and Yang.

Taiji Quan Chan Shou Lian Xi 太極圈纏手練習   Taiji circle sticking hands training. One of the most important trainings in Yang style Taijiquan. This training is used to train listening, understanding, sticking, adhering, connecting, and following. In Chen style, it is called "Silk reeling Jin coiling training" (纏絲勁纏手練習).

Taijiquan (Tai Chi Chuan) 太極拳   A Chinese internal martial style which is based on the theory of Taiji (grand ultimate).

Taipei 台北   The capital city of Taiwan located in the north of Taiwan.

Taipei Xian 台北縣   The county in northern Taiwan.

Taiwan 台灣   An island to the southeast of mainland China. Also known as "Formosa."

Taiwan University 台灣大學   A well-known university located in Taipei, Taiwan.

Taizuquan 太祖拳   A style of Chinese external martial arts.

Tamkang 淡江   Name of a University in Taiwan.

Tamkang College Guoshu Club 淡江國術社   A Chinese martial arts club founded by Dr. Yang when he was studying in Tamkang College.

Ti 提   Means "to lift or to raise."

Ti Shen 提神   Means "to raise up the spirit."

Ting Jin 聽勁   Listening Jin. A special training which uses the skin to feel the opponent's energy and from this feeling to further understand his intention.

Tu 土   Earth. One of the Five Elements.

Tui 退   Retreating backward.

Tui 推   Push. A major technique in Chinese Tui Na (推拿) Qigong massage. When Tui is used in Taijiquan, it is an action of using the palm to push forward, upward, or downward to the opponent's body.

Tui Bu 退步   Means "to step backward." Retreat.

Tui Na 推拿   Means "to push and grab." A category of Chinese massages for healing and injury treatment.

Wang, Zong-Yue 王宗岳 A well known Taijiquan master during the late Qing dynasty. Wang, Zong-Yue wrote many comprehensive Taijiquan documents and is popularly studied by Taijiquan practitioners today.

Wei Qi 衛氣 Protective Qi or Guardian Qi. The Qi at the surface of the body which generates a shield to protect the body from negative external influences such as colds.

Wilson Chen 陳威伸 Dr. Yang, Jwing-Ming's friend.

Wu 午 One of the twelve Terrestrial Branches (i.e., 11 A.M.-1 P.M.).

Wu Bu 五步 Five steppings. They include: forward, backward, left, right, and center.

Wu Xing 五行 Five Phases, including: metal (Jin, 金), wood (Mu, 木), water (Shui, 水), fire (Huo, 火), and earth (Tu, 土).

Wu, Jian-Quan 吳鑑泉 The son of Wu, Quan-You. A second generation practitioner of Wu style Taijiquan.

Wu, Quan-You 吳全佑 The creator of Wu style Taijiquan. Wu, Quan-You learned Taijiquan from Yang, Ban-Hou.

Wudang Mountain 武當山 Located in Hubei Province (湖北省) in China.

Wuji 無極 Means "no extremity."

Wushu 武術 Literally, "martial techniques."

Wuyi 武藝 Literally, "martial arts."

Xia 下 Below, under, or lower.

Xia Dan Tian 下丹田 Lower elixir field. Located in the lower abdomen, it is believed to be the residence of water Qi (Original Qi)(Yuan Qi, 元氣). This cavity in acupuncture is called Qihai (Co-6) (氣海) which means "Qi ocean."

Xia Pan 下盤 The Chinese express the concept of root generated by the legs as the "lower disk." From the thighs to the feet is called Xia Pan (lower disk), the waist area is called "Zhong Pan" (中盤)(middle disk), while the chest and the head are "Shang Pan" (上盤)(top disk)."

Xian Xi 閒隙 Means "leisure gap." It implies that you have extra time for something.

Xiao Lu 小攦 Small rollback.

Xiao Quan 小圈 Means "small circle."

Xin 心 Means "heart." Xin means the mind generated from emotional disturbance.

Xinmen 囟門 A cavity or vital point located on the crown of the head.

Xinzhu Xian 新竹縣 Birthplace of Dr. Yang, Jwing-Ming in Taiwan.

Xu, Xuan-Ping 許宣平 An ancient Taijiquan master who is believed to be one of the possible creators or pioneers of Taijiquan.

Xun 巽 One of the Eight Trigrams.

Yang 仰 Means "bending backward" or "looking upward."

Yang 陽 Too sufficient. One of the two poles. The other is Yin.

Yang Quan 楊拳 Literally, Yang Fist. It means Yang style.

Yang Shen 養氣 Means "nourish the Qi" or "cultivate the Qi in our body."

Yang Wu Di 楊無敵 Means "Unbeatable Yang." A name given to Yang, Lu-Shan by the general public of the time.

Yang, Ban-Hou (1837-1892 A.D.) 楊班侯 Yang, Lu-Shan's second son. Also called Yang, Yu (楊鈺).

Yang, Jian (1839-1917 A.D.) 楊鑑 Yang, Lu-Shan's third son. A second generation practitioner of Yang style Taijiquan. Also named Yang, Jian-Hou (楊健侯) and nicknamed Jing-Hu (鏡湖).

Yang, Jian-Hou (1839-1917 A.D.) 楊健侯 Yang, Lu-Shan's third son. A second generation practitioner of Yang style Taijiquan. Also named Yang, Jian (楊鑑) and nicknamed as Jing-Hu (鏡湖).

Yang, Jwing-Ming 楊俊敏 Author of this book.

Yang, Lu-Shan (1799-1872 A.D.) 楊露禪 The creator of Yang style Taijiquan. He was also known as Fu-Kuai (福魁) or Lu-Shan (祿纏). Born at Yong Nian Xian, Guang Ping County, Hebei Province (河北，廣平府永年縣). When he was young he went to Chen Jia Gou in Henan province (河南陳家溝) to learn Taijiquan from Chen, Chang-Xing (陳長興).

Yang, Qi 楊錡 Yang, Lu-Shan's first son who died at an early age.

Yang, Yu (1837-1892 A.D.) 楊鈺 Yang, Lu-Shan's second son. Also called Ban-Hou (班侯). A second generation practitioner of Yang style Taijiquan.

Yang, Zhao-Peng (1875-1938 A.D.) 楊兆鵬 Yang, Ban-Hou's son. A third generation practitioner of Yang style Taijiquan.

Yang, Zhao-Qing (1883-1936 A.D.) 楊兆清   A third generation practitioner of Yang style Taijiquan. Also named Cheng-Fu (澄甫). He was the first Yang family practitioner who publicized Yang style Taijiquan.

Yang, Zhao-Xiong (1862-1930 A.D.) 楊兆熊   Yang, Jian-Hou's first son. A third generation practitioner of Yang style Taijiquan. Also named Meng-Xiang (夢祥) and later called Shao-Hou (少侯).

Yang, Zhao-Yuan 楊兆元   Yang, Jian-Hou's second son, who died at an early age.

Yang, Zhen-Duo 楊振鐸   Yang, Chen-Fu's third son. One of the fourth generation of Yang style Taijiquan.

Yang, Zhen-Guo 楊振國   Yang, Chen-Fu's fourth son.

Yang, Zhen-Ji 楊振基   Yang, Chen-Fu's second son. One of the fourth generation of Yang style Taijiquan.

Yang, Zhen-Ming 楊振銘   Yang, Chen-Fu's first son. One of the fourth generation of Yang style Taijiquan.

Yang, Zhen-Sheng 楊振聲   Yang, Shao-Hou's son. One of the fourth generation of Yang style Taijiquan.

Yi 意   Wisdom mind. The mind generated from wise judgment.

Yi Jing 易經   *Book of Changes*. A book of divination written during the Zhou Dynasty (1122-255 B.C., 周).

Yin 陰   Deficient. One of the two poles. The other is Yang.

Yin Jin 引勁   The Jin (martial power) of leading.

Yin Jin Luo Kong 引勁落空   Means "to lead the coming Jin into emptiness." It means to neutralize the incoming force.

Yin Li 硬力   Hard muscular force.

You 右   Right.

You Pan 右盼   Means "beware of the right."

Zhan 占   To occupy.

Zhan 粘   Attaching.

Zhan Jin 粘勁   The martial power that is used to attack the opponent's body.

Zhan Qian 瞻前   Gazing to the front.

Zhan Zhuang 站椿   Means "standing on the post." A common terminology for "fundamental stance training."

Zhang Jin 長勁 Growing Jin. One form of the martial power trained in Taijiquan.

Zhang, San-Feng 張三丰 Zhang, San-Feng is credited as the creator of Taijiquan during the Song dynasty in China (960-1127 A.D.)(宋朝).

Zhang, Xiang-San 張祥三 A well-known martial artist in Taiwan during the 1960's.

Zhen 震 One of the Eight Trigrams.

Zhen Ren 真人 Means "real person" or "truthful person." A Daoist aims to be truthful and are therefore called "truthful man."

Zhi Jue Yun Dong 知覺運動 Means the exercise of conscious feeling. This means the practice of feeling sensitivity.

Zhong 中 Centering.

Zhong Dan Tian 中丹田 Middle Dan Tian. Located in the area of the solar plexus, it is the residence of fire Qi.

Zhong Ding 中定 To firm the center.

Zhong Guo Wushu 中國武術 Means Chinese martial arts. Often abbreviated as Wushu.

Zhong Ju 中距 Middle range. A common fighting range in which a kick is able to reach the opponent but not a hand strike.

Zhong Quan 中圈 Middle circle.

Zhong Tu 中土 Means Central Earth. In the Five Phases, the Earth belongs to the center position.

Zhongwan (Co-12) 中脘 The name of an acupuncture cavity at the stomach area. It belongs to the Conceptional vessel.

Zhou 肘 Elbow.

Zhou Jin 肘勁 The martial power generated from the elbow.

Zhua 抓 Means "to grasp" or "to grab."

Zhua Jin 抓筋 Means "to grab the tendons."

Zhuan 轉 Means "to turn around" or " to twist."

Zhuan Jin 轉勁 The martial power of turning.

Zi 子 One of the twelve Terrestrial Branches (i.e., 11 P.M.–1 A.M.).

Zuo 左 Left.

Zuo Gu 左顧 Look to the left or beware of the left.

Zuo Wan 坐腕 Settle down the wrist.

Zuo You 左右 Left and right.

Index

BOOKS FROM YMAA

101 REFLECTIONS ON TAI CHI CHUAN
108 INSIGHTS INTO TAI CHI CHUAN
A WOMAN'S QIGONG GUIDE
ADVANCING IN TAE KWON DO
ANALYSIS OF GENUINE KARATE
ANALYSIS OF GENUINE KARATE 2
ANALYSIS OF SHAOLIN CHIN NA 2ND ED
ANCIENT CHINESE WEAPONS
ART AND SCIENCE OF STAFF FIGHTING
THE ART AND SCIENCE OF SELF-DEFENSE
ART AND SCIENCE OF STICK FIGHTING
ART OF HOJO UNDO
ARTHRITIS RELIEF
BACK PAIN RELIEF
BAGUAZHANG
BRAIN FITNESS
CHIN NA IN GROUND FIGHTING
CHINESE FAST WRESTLING
CHINESE FITNESS
CHINESE TUI NA MASSAGE
COMPLETE MARTIAL ARTIST
COMPREHENSIVE APPLICATIONS OF SHAOLIN CHIN NA
CONFLICT COMMUNICATION
DAO DE JING: A QIGONG INTERPRETATION
DAO IN ACTION
DEFENSIVE TACTICS
DIRTY GROUND
DR. WU'S HEAD MASSAGE
ESSENCE OF SHAOLIN WHITE CRANE
EXPLORING TAI CHI
FACING VIOLENCE
FIGHT LIKE A PHYSICIST
THE FIGHTER'S BODY
FIGHTER'S FACT BOOK 1&2
FIGHTING THE PAIN RESISTANT ATTACKER
FIRST DEFENSE
FORCE DECISIONS: A CITIZENS GUIDE
INSIDE TAI CHI
JUDO ADVANTAGE
JUJI GATAME ENCYCLOPEDIA
KARATE SCIENCE
KEPPAN
KRAV MAGA COMBATIVES
KRAV MAGA FUNDAMENTAL STRATEGIES
KRAV MAGA PROFESSIONAL TACTICS
KRAV MAGA WEAPON DEFENSES
LITTLE BLACK BOOK OF VIOLENCE
LIUHEBAFA FIVE CHARACTER SECRETS
MARTIAL ARTS OF VIETNAM
MARTIAL ARTS INSTRUCTION
MARTIAL WAY AND ITS VIRTUES
MEDITATIONS ON VIOLENCE
MERIDIAN QIGONG EXERCISES
MINDFUL EXERCISE
MIND INSIDE TAI CHI
MIND INSIDE YANG STYLE TAI CHI CHUAN
NORTHERN SHAOLIN SWORD
OKINAWA'S COMPLETE KARATE SYSTEM: ISSHIN RYU
PRINCIPLES OF TRADITIONAL CHINESE MEDICINE
PROTECTOR ETHIC
QIGONG FOR HEALTH & MARTIAL ARTS
QIGONG FOR TREATING COMMON AILMENTS

QIGONG MASSAGE
QIGONG MEDITATION: EMBRYONIC BREATHING
QIGONG GRAND CIRCULATION
QIGONG MEDITATION: SMALL CIRCULATION
QIGONG, THE SECRET OF YOUTH: DA MO'S CLASSICS
ROOT OF CHINESE QIGONG
SAMBO ENCYCLOPEDIA
SCALING FORCE
SELF-DEFENSE FOR WOMEN
SHIN GI TAI: KARATE TRAINING
SIMPLE CHINESE MEDICINE
SIMPLE QIGONG EXERCISES FOR HEALTH, 3RD ED.
SIMPLIFIED TAI CHI CHUAN, 2ND ED.
SOLO TRAINING 1&2
SPOTTING DANGER BEFORE IT SPOTS YOU
SPOTTING DANGER BEFORE IT SPOTS YOUR KIDS
SPOTTING DANGER BEFORE IT SPOTS YOUR TEENS
SPOTTING DANGER FOR TRAVELERS
SUMO FOR MIXED MARTIAL ARTS
SUNRISE TAI CHI
SURVIVING ARMED ASSAULTS
TAE KWON DO: THE KOREAN MARTIAL ART
TAEKWONDO BLACK BELT POOMSAE
TAEKWONDO: A PATH TO EXCELLENCE
TAEKWONDO: ANCIENT WISDOM
TAEKWONDO: DEFENSE AGAINST WEAPONS
TAEKWONDO: SPIRIT AND PRACTICE
TAI CHI BALL QIGONG: FOR HEALTH AND MARTIAL ARTS
TAI CHI BALL QIGONG
THE TAI CHI BOOK
TAI CHI CHIN NA
TAI CHI CHUAN CLASSICAL YANG STYLE
TAI CHI CHUAN MARTIAL APPLICATIONS
TAI CHI CHUAN MARTIAL POWER
TAI CHI CONCEPTS AND EXPERIMENTS
TAI CHI DYNAMICS
TAI CHI FOR DEPRESSION
TAI CHI IN 10 WEEKS
TAI CHI PUSH HANDS
TAI CHI QIGONG
TAI CHI SECRETS OF THE ANCIENT MASTERS
TAI CHI SECRETS OF THE WU & LI STYLES
TAI CHI SECRETS OF THE WU STYLE
TAI CHI SECRETS OF THE YANG STYLE
TAI CHI SWORD: CLASSICAL YANG STYLE
TAI CHI SWORD FOR BEGINNERS
TAI CHI WALKING
TAI CHI CHUAN THEORY OF DR. YANG, JWING-MING
FIGHTING ARTS
TRADITIONAL CHINESE HEALTH SECRETS
TRADITIONAL TAEKWONDO
TRAINING FOR SUDDEN VIOLENCE
TRIANGLE HOLD ENCYCLOPEDIA
TRUE WELLNESS SERIES (MIND, HEART, GUT)
WARRIOR'S MANIFESTO
WAY OF KATA
WAY OF SANCHIN KATA
WAY TO BLACK BELT
WESTERN HERBS FOR MARTIAL ARTISTS
WILD GOOSE QIGONG
WING CHUN IN-DEPTH
WINNING FIGHTS
XINGYIQUAN

AND MANY MORE . . .

VIDEOS FROM YMAA

AND MANY MORE . . .

more products available from . . .

YMAA Publication Center, Inc.   楊氏東方文化出版中心

1-800-669-8892 • info@ymaa.com • www.ymaa.com

YMAA
PUBLICATION CENTER

www.ingramcontent.com/pod-product-compliance
Lightning Source LLC
Chambersburg PA
CBHW062008090426
42811CB00005B/789